SO MUCH MORE THAN A HEADACHE

LITERATURE AND MEDICINE
Michael Blackie, Editor • Carol Donley and Martin Kohn, Founding Editors

So Much More Than
a Headache

Understanding Migraine
through Literature

Edited by

KATHLEEN J. O'SHEA

THE KENT STATE UNIVERSITY PRESS

Kent, Ohio

© 2020 by The Kent State University Press, Kent, Ohio 44242
ALL RIGHTS RESERVED
Library of Congress Catalog Number 2020000701
ISBN 978-1-60635-403-2
Manufactured in the United States of America

LIBRARY OF CONGRESS CATALOGING-IN-PUBLICATION DATA
Names: O'Shea, Kathleen J., editor.
Title: So much more than a headache : understanding migraine through literature /
        edited by Kathleen J. O'Shea.
Description: Kent, Ohio : The Kent State University Press, 2020. | Series: Literature and
        medicine series
Identifiers: LCCN 2020000701 (print) | LCCN 2020000702 (ebook) | ISBN
        9781606354032 (paperback) | ISBN 9781631014178 (ebook) | ISBN
        9781631014185 (pdf)
Subjects: LCSH: Migraine--Popular works.
Classification: LCC RC392 .S5755 2050 (print) | LCC RC392 (ebook) | DDC
        616.8/4912--dc23
LC record available at https://lccn.loc.gov/2020000701
LC ebook record available at https://lccn.loc.gov/2020000702

24 23 22 21 20   5 4 3 2 1

For Dr. Joseph Mann, who has always listened, encouraged, and found another way, and who has helped me through the worst and taught me the most—my doctor, mentor, and friend

Contents

PART V: WHEN IT'S GONE . . .

Preface

This collection of imaginative works by fiction writers, poets, and essayists ranging over five centuries, some famous, some not, but most of them migraine sufferers themselves, is directed, first of all, but not solely to, those who suffer migraine. Here, they will find the companionship of other migraine sufferers who can perhaps better express what they have grappled to put into words for themselves and for others.

Those others for whom this anthology is intended include medical practitioners, who may or not be specialists in migraines but also, importantly, those family members and friends who observe their suffering but want and need to understand better this disease.

Those who employ or work with migraine sufferers can benefit from better understanding the full range of the illness, one that, to so many, can appear invisible. In a classroom setting, instructors and students can benefit by reading and discussing any common text but in this case works concentrated on a very specific range of experience that is the literature of illness.

MY PERSPECTIVE AS EDITOR

As a forty-two-year migraineur, I need to take stock. At fifty-six, I find myself in a new, frightening place: my superb headache specialist for years has retired, and I realize now more than ever how much I relied not only on his regular and kind care but on his constant reassurance that new medications and treatment options, now designed specifically for migraine, were on the horizon.

I decided, at a time when migraine had seemingly taken residence (three months) with a day here and there of relief, I needed to do something positive and productive with this significant dimension of my life. Rather than sinking into the pain, dwelling on what I cannot do, feel, or experience, I found myself turning to what always consoles, informs, and guides me—literature.

Many self-help books today make claims, offer solutions, and outline the ways by which migraineurs can eradicate this very mind-set, can take us "out of ourselves," work to get off all of our medications—often just through more exercise, better eating, and meditation. While these activities are generally good for all of us, what lies within many such texts is an implicit suggestion that what we really need is to shift our attitude that both the "headaches" and the roles they play in our lives are entirely within our control to manage or even cure. Some of these books' titles alone—*You Can Heal Your Life* or *Mind over Migraine*—leave me, at best, shaking my head—more evidence that there remains so much ignorance about this disease. The truth is, most of the general public still see migraine as "only a headache," rather than the complex brain disease we now know it is.

Many sufferers often seek support and understanding through migraine support groups and, more recently, blogging. The *New York Times* ran an excellent regular column/blog on migraine in 2008, featuring columns by established writers, including Siri Hustvedt and Paula Kamen. These articles, one of which is included in this anthology, provide patient and expert perspectives on episodic and chronic migraine. These avenues are certainly valuable, but I suggest that literature best captures the essence of pain and suffering, subjectively and imaginatively.

As a professor of literature for thirty-two years, I often work with students who have had little or no experience in reading and appreciating literature. Initially, some even have disdain for the subject. Many of these students have also lived with significant pain of all kinds; they have life stories that are unimaginable. I love teaching literature when these students discover that first piece of poetry, that first short story or novel that shows them they are not alone, that someone else has felt what they have, that someone does "get it." At that point, I know they're hooked.

I hope to demonstrate through this collection that, indeed, literature, like all of the arts, offers to its reader subjective and imaginative experiences that we often find difficult to describe, at least in ways that aren't clinical and objective. Those of us who live with migraine in all of its forms crave having someone understand, truly understand, what we live with—the often excruciating pain we think no one else could possibly have endured—the losses, loneliness, and sacrifices directly and indirectly caused by this disease. The works in this anthology will appeal to friends and family who want to better comprehend the extensive range of symptoms, the effects of medications, and the emotional struggle that envelops their loved one throughout the migraine cycle.

Literature captures the essence of all forms of joy and pain, and readers of all ages and backgrounds connect with grief and struggle. Sometimes, it helps us confront fear, hopelessness, and weariness. It cracks open the door on subjects we have buried, rationalized about, or hidden from. It tackles the gray areas of life, grappling with subjects that aren't black and white, often leaving us in inevitable ambiguity rather than clear resolution.

As with literature, this state of ambiguity is where many migraineurs find themselves. There are no simple solutions for migraine and its complexity of pain and suffering; there is no "cure." The "answers" come in fits and spurts through the right combinations of treatments, lifestyle, and support. Like my students' struggles, which are complex and multilayered, so is life with migraine, but literature speaks to all; it does so in a way that reaches us viscerally.

Medical professionals must cope with the individuality of each migraineur's experience; no two migraine patients are the same. The literature here demonstrates this disparity and breadth of each person's experience; some writers focus on the aura, with amazement in some cases and fear in others. Some writers focus on the range of symptoms in each phase of the cycle, while others capture the seemingly endless search for effective treatment. Practitioners want and need to recognize the variability of the patients with whom they work.

Kevin Young, in his introduction to the anthology *The Art of Losing*, begins: "I have begun to believe in, and even to preach, a poetry of necessity . . . the best poems, it seems to me, evince their origins in the need to speak, or to write; to render a complex fate simply; to render chaos as chaos. . . . A poem must be willing to be unwilled, beckoned by need."[1] In writing about the healing force of poetry, poet Mary Oliver argues, "poetry is a life-cherishing force. For poems are not words, after all, but fires for the cold, ropes let down to the lost, something as necessary as bread in the pockets of the hungry. Yes indeed."[2]

Renowned psychologists, researchers, and fiction writers, including Virginia Woolf, have argued that pain is extremely difficult to characterize, to describe in words. Elaine Scarry's compelling argument in *The Body in Pain: The Making and Unmaking of the World* suggests that "Whatever pain achieves, it achieves in part through its unsharability, and it ensures this unsharability through its resistance to language."[3] She further suggests that "physical pain—unlike any other state of consciousness—has no referential content . . . because the existing vocabulary for pain contains only a small handful of adjectives, one passes through direct descriptions very quickly," resulting in common "as if" constructions.[4] While I concede that "the exceptional character of pain when compared to all of our other interior states" often renders us silent, I argue through this collection that literature *can* capture the authentic voice and language in ways objective texts cannot.

Think about when the migraineur is asked to describe his or her "headache" to doctors, friends, and family: "It feels as if someone has my head in a vise . . . It feels like shooting pain through my eye . . . It's as if someone sucked out all the life in me." These metaphors or comparisons, while somewhat descriptive, are not really part of the experience either, as Scarry points out.

Virginia Woolf, the great twentieth-century novelist and a migraineur herself, claims that "English, which can express the thoughts of Hamlet and the tragedy of Lear has no words for the shiver or the headache. . . . The merest school girl when she falls in love has Shakespeare or Keats to speak her mind for her, but let a sufferer try to describe a pain in his head to a doctor and language at once runs dry."[5]

While we are in pain, language often fails us, that's true. How many times have migraineurs been asked to rate on a scale of "one to ten" their pain level and been frustrated, even exasperated, by the question, wondering, "Does that mean my actual throbbing migraine/headache, or this migraine relative to other migraine headache events I've had? . . . Isn't my scale of pain likely different from someone who hasn't had migraine for a number of years? . . . How does this scale address the multitude of symptoms that accompany migraine, those that may leave me 'functional' but at such a cost? Does the scale measure that?"

We can let literature speak for us; it does not measure the experience, but, instead, it *illustrates* responses to all of these questions and more.

Adam Smith, an eighteenth-century writer, describes pain and suffering from the perspective of those who are feeling it *and* those observing:

> As we have no immediate experience of what other men feel, we can form no idea of the manner in which they are affected but by conceiving what we ourselves should feel in the like situation. . . . By the imagination we place ourselves in his situation, we conceive ourselves enduring all the same torments, we enter as it were into his body, and become in some measure the same person with him.[6]

Through the discovery of literature we develop empathy. Convincingly, Martha Stoddard Holmes and Tod Chambers in their essay "Thinking through Pain" argue that "expressed pain, relieved pain, remembered pain's reliance on the very representation that sometimes eludes it has thus opened a particular space for the humanities."[7] The author of the text, who may well be the sufferer, must also be the observer, who can distance himself or herself enough to channel the suffering into aesthetic, social, and sometimes political themes. Why, then, historically, has there been relatively little great literature about chronic illness and pain?

In 1926, poet and critic T. S. Eliot commissioned novelist Virginia Woolf to write an essay "On Being Ill" for the British literary magazine the *Criterion* shortly after Woolf suffered a nervous breakdown. Her central concern in the piece is why illness is not an integral theme of literature:

> Considering how common illness is, how tremendous the spiritual change that it brings, how astonishing, when the lights of health go down, the undiscovered countries that are then disclosed, what wastes and deserts of the soul a slight attack of influenza brings to light, what precipices and lawns sprinkled with bright flowers a little rise of temperature reveals . . . it becomes strange indeed that illness has not taken its place with love, battle, and jealousy among the prime themes of literature.[8]

This poignant passage articulates the position that the subject of chronic illness needs to become a more integral part of our literary canon, and, fortunately, we do see this trend shifting. The humanities and more recently migraine/headache specialists and neurologists are recognizing this necessity, in part, because of the role narrative plays in illness and pain. Dr. Judy Segal, professor and researcher on rhetorical elements in public discourse on pain, declares, "narrative . . . gives meaning and texture and humanity."[9]

In recent decades there has been an explosion of course work, books, and programming on literature and medicine. In fact, many of the best medical universities in the country have fully developed programs in medicine and the humanities. Medicine & the Muse is the home for the arts and humanities at the Stanford University Medical School, with programs that integrate the arts and humanities into medical education and medical practice. Courses like the Nature of Illness at the University Colorado Health Sciences Center acknowledge the idea that illness, particularly the voice and experience of the patient, is often made silent or at least diminished in medical practice and, therefore, work with their students to better understand the subjective element of pain and suffering.

Wonderful databases and websites like *Project Muse* provide tremendous links among the medical fields and the broader humanities. John Hopkins University Press's *Literature and Medicine* journal has been featuring prominent writers and scholars grappling with different themes related to illness and pain since 1982.

This anthology will afford medical students and their professors a substantive tool to teach empathy and compassion, especially in an age when technology in the doctor's office pulls doctors and patients farther and farther apart.

THE MIGRAINE AND NARRATIVE

Not all literature employs narrative, and some illnesses are sudden and its onset to its resolution happens very quickly. But migraine shares with fiction, drama, and some kinds of poetry the device of narrative—that is, a distinctive beginning, middle, and end. Each migraine has its own duration, and during the life of a migraineur he or she can designate and remember all too vividly the first migraine and how the disease has ramified in its symptoms and intensity. True enough, there are often cycles in migraine—there is not just one beginning, middle, and end, but this cyclicality is often a hallmark of many kinds of literature, just as it is of migraine.

Migraineurs will recall their first appointment with each doctor they have seen for migraine, the time they are asked to give their *history:* "Well, I had my first migraine when I was fourteen, and then . . . and then . . . and now . . ." When we want to better understand the time line of an illness, we create narrative; we become storytellers. When thinking about a personal narrative history of migraine, though, we start to realize that the story is not linear; it cannot be expressed in a straight line. In fact, the "story line" is circuitous. It turns back on itself, and then goes in new directions, before it brings us to the present.

For many, particularly chronic migraineurs, the migraine cycle itself is at least as circuitous. It often starts with the Prodromal Phase, the warning signs that an attack is likely. Such signs can include uncontrollable yawning, extreme fatigue, hypersensitivity to sound and/or light, cravings, and other visceral symptoms such as pain in the deep muscles of the neck that, with one strong wrong movement, can set off a full-blown attack. Before an actual headache, others experience an "aura," an electrical activation of the brain that is an immediate portent of a migraine.

Here's where the narrative gets complicated. With personal knowledge of such early signs, migraineurs know they are supposed to take medications for an acute attack early, with the hope of warding off the worst. Sometimes, the narrative slows down here, as we question whether it's too early, whether we want to use the precious medications and injections, since we don't want to run out before insurance will cover them again. If a full-blown attack does occur, the narrative slows down even more, for hours or days, sometimes weeks, before there's any sign of relief—time seems to stop.

The narrative then takes a turn. Maybe the headache and accompanying symptoms lift completely, and then the narrative can come to a slow ending, as you enter the Postdrome Phase. We now cope with the "hangover feeling," moving through the day feeling like our head weighs one ton on our neck. We are overwhelmingly fatigued, still experiencing problems with cognitive functions and focus. Word drops and an overall feeling of not being well pervade.

For many chronic migraineurs, the movement of the narrative takes numerous twists and turns. The migraine, after days of incapacitation, eventually lifts enough for us to "function," and this part of the journey can be interminable. This lower (albeit constant) level of pain, the inability to focus, the cognitive problems (blanks, difficulty coming up with words), the general feeling of being unwell and fuzzy, and the lack of stamina to do any more than is absolutely necessary can go on for weeks or months before the cycle either morphs back into a full-blown attack, maybe giving us one day of feeling "pretty good" before reverting at any time.

Even after the migraine event has passed, there remains the last phase of the cycle, the Postdrome, leaving many with a "migraine hangover." This phase, for some, leaves a general feeling of being "wiped out" or "run over by a truck," extremely fatigued and barely able to hold up their heads. For some, though, the end of the cycle leaves them with a state of "migraine euphoria," knowing immediately that everything associated with the attack/cycle has somehow "lifted" out of their body, that indescribable lightness; they can appreciate life again.

However, before long, the fear sets in as they question how long this respite will last, wondering if they can *ever* go through that ordeal again. This story is finished, perhaps for a day, or a week, or, with the right support systems in place, even months, before a variation of the next narrative begins anew.

This circuitous path is, of course, affected by the medical treatment we have along the way—experimenting with numerous preventative, acute, and rescue medications and trips to see our neurologist or headache specialist for nerve blocks, Botox, injections, IV medications, and, ultimately, brand-new developments in research and treatments. This, then, is our unique migraine narrative.

The narrative device is one of the key elements you'll find in many of the works in this anthology. This collection is, of course, by no means exhaustive, but it examines many themes related to migraine. The sections are organized according to several recognizable themes: "What It Feels Like," "What People Don't See: The Invisibility of Migraine," "It's Just a Headache?," "It's a Lifelong, Full-Time Job," and "When It's Gone . . ." Readers will notice that some works touch on *several* of the themes and, therefore, could have been placed in other parts. While true, my intent is to emphasize certain aspects of an individual work, recognizing its broader ability to speak to many themes and audiences.

THE OVERALL ORGANIZATION OF THIS ANTHOLOGY

The order of the parts has a multilayered organizational structure. First, beginning and ending the book with two outstanding essays that speak to *all* of the themes in the book provides a solid structural and aesthetic framework. How do we discover the literature that will speak to us? Sometimes, it discovers us. Preparing to teach my first composition class as a graduate student in 1985, I opened the textbook I'd be using for the course, and the first essay was "In Bed," by the widely acclaimed writer Joan Didion. I found this essay, published in 1984, immediately jarring in its genuine grasp of what I experienced with migraine. It authoritatively provides a narrative of shifting voices, something migraineurs live with every day. Didion uses her own voice to exquisitely describe the migraine experience, but she also shifts to society's general, often ignorant voice in response to migraine.

At first, she internalizes these external voices: "For I had no brain tumor, or eyestrain, no high blood pressure, nothing wrong with me at all. I simply had migraine headaches."[10] Didion comes about as close to capturing the pain and its effects on the mind and body as any work written. This work, which could have been excerpted for any of the parts in this anthology, put its lasting mark on migraine narrative; therefore, I begin with this piece in its entirety.

The disease is sometimes invisible, often making sufferers feel invisible: "Why not take a couple of aspirin" or "I have headaches too."[11] Eventually, Didion rejects these voices and transforms the migraine into something with which she acknowledges she has a relationship: "I have learned now to live with it. . . . We have reached a certain understanding, my migraine and I."[12]

This essay struck a number of chords with me—she "gets it," not just the quality and experience of the headache itself but the numerous other aspects of the disease, which are too often invisible to others. She also exquisitely captures the overwhelming fear with each migraine that "this one" will be endless, will never "lift" entirely.

The anthology concludes with Anna Leahy's essay, "Half-Skull Days," which, like Didion's, richly captures each of the five themes in the book and serves beautifully as a touchstone for the anthology's overarching ideas:

> The staved-off migraine's disorientation has left me aware of my own incoherence, my inability to track time accurately or to guess what I might say next, or not be able to say. When I couldn't think of the word *scale,* upon which I had slammed my toe and made a racket in the bathroom only moments before, I pantomimed stepping onto the scale and looking down to see my weight. But even my husband is not used to this sort of communication and shrugged; at least he was no longer worried that I'd injured myself. I would not call what I felt in this semi-articulate moment *pain,* but I was suffering. Every bit of coherence I mustered took great effort, when lucidity is usually taken for granted, like breathing.[13]

Beginning with the experience itself and concluding with its relief (albeit temporary) gives the book some linear sense—this horror will end.

However, the temporary nature of the migraine's departure and its natural return to the essence of the experience described in part I: "What It Feels Like" parallels the circuitous nature of migraine as disease.

The great poet Emily Dickinson confronts such suffering:

> Pain has an element of blank;
> It cannot recollect
> when it began, or if there were
> a day when it was not[14]

Dickinson, in the grip of pain herself, understands that it's difficult to distinguish past, present, and future in terms of the pain; our lives and identities become consumed by pain.

Such writers also understand that in the midst of migraine, the fact that the headache itself won't be fatal does not always seem positive. These writers capture the truthful ambivalence the sufferer sometimes feels about surviving it. As critic Lucy Ferris writes, "I enter Dickinson's world; no memory of anything before the pain, no future without it. I am afraid of death. Yet, if someone in authority were to say to me, in the midst of the four worst days, 'This is the shape of the rest of your life,' I would put a bullet in to my brain without thinking twice about it."[15]

The second and third parts—"What People Don't See: The Invisibility of Migraine" and "It's Just a Headache?"—follow the stigma and misunderstandings involving the disease, leading us into the multitude of treatments, the lifetime of struggles, and the weariness that come with living with chronic illness, leading us into part IV, "It's a Lifelong, Full-Time Job," which focuses on the multitude of treatments, lifetime of struggles, and the weariness from living for years with chronic illness.

The last part of the book, "When It's Gone . . . ," takes us to the "migraine hangover" many experience, as well as the "migraine euphoria" others feel.

While most of this collection focuses on the costs and sacrifices of living with migraine—as well as the larger impacts the disease brings its sufferers, their doctors, friends, family, and employers—this last part brings us closer to the incredible advancements recently available, with several more on the near horizon. Calcitonin gene-related peptide (CGRP) inhibitors, now available to the public, and the Cefaly device, used for acute attacks and as a preventative treatment, are some of the first truly revolutionary treatments specifically targeted for migraine disease. Some studies suggest these treatments can give our lives back to many of us.

And so we come back to the idea of the narrative, the journey as an archetype in literature—whether the life journey or, in our case, the migraine journey—the obstacles we face, the constant struggles, most never seen by others, but also the hope of something in the near future that will be our chalice on reaching our goal, after facing and surmounting so much.

My interest in putting together this anthology is, then, manifold: I want to champion the power and value of great literature to speak in ways that people experiencing migraine feel they cannot. I want to demonstrate the beauty of poetry, drama, essay, and fiction to capture the essence of migraine, even as patients are evolving in their own understanding and treatment. I want to reach those who have not experienced migraine firsthand to experience it through a persona, to see the ways in which the disease takes hold of a person's (and family's) entire life.

For those studying medicine, pain, and literature, my hope is that this collection will offer what the scales, whether the "McGill Pain Questionnaire" or the "Rate My Pain" form in the typical waiting room, cannot. These forms migraineurs fill out so routinely cannot capture pain, the physical and psychological effects of headache, and the multitude of side effects patients live with from many preventative, acute, and rescue medications—the individual narrative.

My hope is that this collection offers migraineurs some solace in knowing they are not alone, some comfort when they feel weak and helpless in their pain, some assurance that so many others have traveled their path or one close to it, and, ultimately, some recognition of the moments of appreciation they feel when experiencing "time off" from the disease.

If migraineurs feel less alone and more certain of shared experience, they will also greatly benefit from their loved ones, employers, and medical professionals having a place to turn to better understand the experience of migraine, its many manifestations, and the diverse paths it takes.

NOTES

1. Kevin Young, *The Art of Losing: Poems of Grief & Healing* (New York: Bloomsbury, 2013), xv.
2. Mary Oliver, *A Poetry Handbook* (New York: Harcourt Brace, 1994), 122.
3. Elaine Scarry, *The Body in Pain: The Making and Unmaking of the World* (New York: Oxford Univ. Press, 1985), 4.
4. Scarry, *The Body in Pain,* 5, 15.
5. Virginia Woolf, "On Illness," in *On Being Ill* (Ashfield, MA: Paris Press, 2002), 4.
6. Adam Smith, *The Theory of Moral Sentiments,* Glasgow Edition of the *Works and Correspondence of Adam Smith,* ed. D. D. Raphael and A. L. Macfie (Indianapolis, IN: Liberty Fund, 1982), 9.
7. Martha Stoddard Homes and Tod Chambers, "Thinking through Pain," *Literature and Medicine* 18, no. 1 (2005): 135.
8. Woolf, "On Illness," 3.
9. Judy Z. Segal, *Health and the Rhetoric of Medicine* (Carbondale: Southern Illinois Univ. Press, 2008), https://muse.jhu.edu/book/21758ER.
10. Joan Didion, "In Bed," in *The White Album* (New York: Farrar, Strauss, and Giroux, 1979), 68.
11. Didion, "In Bed," 68.
12. Didion, 68.
13. Anna Leahy, "Half-Skull Days," *The Pinch* (Spring 2012): 240.
14. Emily Dickinson, "Pain Has an Element of Blank," in *The Poems of Emily Dickinson,* ed. Thomas H. Johnson (Cambridge, MA: Harvard Univ. Press, 1955), lines 1–4.
15. Lucy Ferriss, "Meditation on Pain," *Prairie Schooner* 91, no. 2 (Summer 2017): 111.

Acknowledgments

I am grateful for the loving support of my husband Ed, who knows firsthand what it's like to live with and support a chronic migraineur and who has worked by my side with this project since its inception.

Of course, my dear parents Fred and Joy Goodrich started my migraine journey with me when I was only fourteen and have remained to this day my staunchest advocates and unwavering supporters.

My dear friend Mary Ann always "gets it," always knows how best to help, listen, and be there for the writing of this book and with everything else.

My friend Joan has worked tirelessly to assist me with the compiling and editing of this book and has always stood by me with unwavering friendship. My "bud" and many other colleagues/friends hold me up and help me through many hard migraine times and have lovingly encouraged me with this project from the beginning.

Frederick Godley, MD, and president of the Association of Migraine Disorders, demonstrated support early on in the project, giving me generous financial support that was crucial to this project moving forward. I'm so very grateful for his belief in me and this book.

In addition to Dr. Joseph Mann, my longtime headache specialist, Lesley Lange, DC, and Jenni Tuller, PT, have for so many years made up my faithful, dedicated, and compassionate migraine medical team; I have been blessed with all of them.

Special thanks to the Kent State University Press, specifically William Underwood, acquiring editor; Susan Wadsworth-Booth, director; Mary Young, managing editor; and Michael Blackie, Literature and Medicine series editor, for their belief in the importance of this book and their ready assistance from the original proposal to the final product. Thanks, too, to Valerie Ahwee, who was helpful and personable in all her assistance.

In Bed

JOAN DIDION

THREE, FOUR, sometimes five times a month, I spend the day in bed with a migraine headache, insensible to the world around me. Almost every day of every month, between these attacks, I feel the sudden irrational irritation and the flush of blood into the cerebral arteries which tell me that migraine is on its way, and I take certain drugs to avert its arrival. If I did not take the drugs, I would be able to function perhaps one day in four. The physiological error called migraine is, in brief, central to the given of my life. When I was 15, 16, even 25, I used to think that I could rid myself of this error by simply denying it, character over chemistry. "Do you have headaches *sometimes? frequently? never?*" the application forms would demand. "Check one." Wary of the trap, wanting whatever it was that the successful circumnavigation of that particular form could bring (a job, a scholarship, the respect of mankind and the grace of God), I would check one. "*Sometimes,*" I would lie. That in fact I spent one or two days a week almost unconscious with pain seemed a shameful secret, evidence not merely of some chemical inferiority but of all my bad attitudes, unpleasant tempers, wrongthink.

For I had no brain tumor, no eyestrain, no high blood pressure, nothing wrong with me at all: I simply had migraine headaches, and migraine headaches were, as everyone who did not have them knew, imaginary. I fought migraine then, ignored the warnings it sent, went to school and later to work in spite of it, sat through lectures in Middle English and presentations to advertisers with involuntary tears running down the right side of my face, threw up in washrooms, stumbled home by instinct, emptied ice trays onto my bed and tried to freeze the pain in my right temple, wished only for a neurosurgeon who would do a lobotomy on house call, and cursed my imagination.

It was a long time before I began thinking mechanistically enough to accept migraine for what it was: something with which I would be living, the way some people live with diabetes. Migraine is something more than the fancy of a neurotic imagination. It is an essentially hereditary complex of symptoms, the most frequently noted but by no means the most unpleasant of which is a vascular headache of blinding severity, suffered by a surprising number of women, a fair number of men (Thomas Jefferson had migraine, and so did Ulysses S. Grant, the day he accepted Lee's surrender), and by some unfortunate children as young as two years old. (I had my first when I was eight. It came on during a fire drill at the Columbia School in Colorado Springs, Colorado. I was taken first home and then to the infirmary at Peterson Field, where my father was stationed. The Air Corps doctor prescribed an enema.) Almost anything can trigger a specific attack of migraine: stress, allergy, fatigue, an abrupt change in barometric pressure, a contretemps over a parking ticket. A flashing light. A fire drill. One inherits, of course, only the predisposition. In other words I spent yesterday in bed with a headache not merely because of my bad attitudes, unpleasant tempers and wrongthink, but because both my grandmothers had migraine, my father has migraine and my mother has migraine.

No one knows precisely what it is that is inherited. The chemistry of migraine, however, seems to have some connection with the nerve hormone named serotonin, which is naturally present in the brain. The amount of serotonin in the blood falls sharply at the onset of migraine, and one migraine drug, methysergide, or Sansert, seems to have some effect on serotonin. Methysergide is a derivative of lysergic acid (in fact Sandoz Pharmaceuticals first synthesized LSD-25 while looking for a migraine cure), and its use is hemmed about with so many contraindications and side effects that most doctors prescribe it only in the most incapacitating cases. Methysergide, when it is prescribed, is taken daily, as a preventive; another preventive which works for some people is old-fashioned ergotamine tartrate, which helps to constrict the swelling blood vessels during the "aura," the period which in most cases precedes the actual headache.

Once an attack is under way, however, no drug touches it. Migraine gives some people mild hallucinations, temporarily blinds others, shows up not only as a headache but as a gastrointestinal disturbance, a painful sensitivity to all sensory stimuli, an abrupt overpowering fatigue, a strokelike aphasia, and a crippling inability to make even the most routine connections. When I am in a migraine aura (for some people the aura lasts fifteen minutes, for others several hours), I will drive through red lights, lose the house keys, spill whatever I am holding, lose the ability to focus my eyes or frame coherent sentences, and generally give the appearance of being on drugs, or drunk. The actual headache, when it comes, brings with it chills, sweating, nausea, a debility that seems to stretch the very limits of endurance. That no one dies of migraine seems, to someone deep into an attack, an ambiguous blessing.

My husband also has migraine, which is unfortunate for him but fortunate for me: perhaps nothing so tends to prolong an attack as the accusing eye of someone who has never had a headache. "Why not take a couple of aspirin," the unafflicted will say from the doorway, or "I'd have a headache, too, spending a beautiful day like this inside with all the shades drawn." All of us who have migraine suffer not only from the attacks themselves but from this common conviction that we are perversely refusing to cure ourselves by taking a couple of aspirin, that we are making ourselves sick, that we "bring it on ourselves." And in the most immediate sense, the sense of why we have a headache this Tuesday and not last Thursday, of course we often do. There certainly is what doctors call a "migraine personality," and that personality tends to be ambitious, inward, intolerant of error, rather rigidly organized, perfectionist. "You don't look like a migraine personality," a doctor once said to me. "Your hair's messy. But I suppose you're a compulsive housekeeper." Actually, my house is kept even more negligently than my hair, but the doctor was right nonetheless: perfectionism can also take the form of spending most of a week writing and rewriting and not writing a single paragraph.

But not all perfectionists have migraine, and not all migrainous people have migraine personalities. We do not escape heredity. I have tried in most of the available ways to escape my own migrainous heredity (at one point I learned to give myself two daily injections of histamine with a hypodermic needle, even though the needle so frightened me that I had to close my eyes when I did it), but I still have migraine. And I have learned now to live with it, learned when to expect it, how to outwit it, even how to regard it, when it does come, as more friend than lodger. We have reached a certain understanding, my migraine and I. It never comes when I am in real trouble. Tell me that my house is burned down, my husband has left me, that there is gunfighting in the streets and panic in the banks, and I will not respond by getting a headache. It comes instead when I am fighting not an open but a guerrilla war with my own life, during weeks of small household confusions, lost laundry, unhappy help, canceled appointments, on days when the telephone rings too much and I get no work done and the wind is coming up. On days like that my friend comes uninvited.

And once it comes, now that I am wise in its ways, I no longer fight it. I lie down and let it happen. At first every small apprehension is magnified, every anxiety a pounding terror. Then the pain comes, and I concentrate only on that. Right there is the usefulness of migraine, there in that imposed yoga, the concentration on the pain. For when the pain recedes, ten or twelve hours later, everything goes with it, all the hidden resentments, all the vain anxieties. The migraine has acted as a circuit breaker, and the fuses have emerged intact. There is a pleasant convalescent euphoria. I open the windows and feel the air, eat gratefully, sleep well. I notice the particular nature of a flower in a glass on the stair landing. I count my blessings.

PART I

What It Feels Like

Introduction

If you are reading this anthology as a migraine sufferer, you will be acutely interested in the works in this part, which describe so directly and powerfully the symptoms and condition, the phases and cycle of the total migraine experience. As we now know, this disease varies greatly among those who share it. While some migraineurs first experience more obvious warning signs such as significant neck pain prior to the actual "headache," still others start the cycle with lesser-known warnings—excessive yawning, for instance; heightened sensitivity to sounds, light, and smells; and trouble communicating and putting sentences together. What most do share, then, is some sort of "warning," known as the Prodromal Phase of a migraine attack. For others, the classic "aura" (visual experience) immediately precedes the actual headache attack.

The first works in this part focus around this early phase of the cycle. Several works that follow capture the essence, the visceral experience of the actual migraine attack, the kind of intense pain that has long been determined to be so difficult to capture in words.

Jean Hanson's "The Lightning in My Eyes" and Claudia Emerson's poem "Migraine: Aura and Aftermath" speak to the 20 percent of migraineurs who experience the aura prior to a migraine attack. Linda Pastan's "Migraine" immediately immerses us with the fractured sensory experience:

Ambushed by
pins and needles
of light . . . by jagged

voices . . . by strobes . . .[1]

The "headache" phase, where most suffer with extraordinary pain, varies in length from hours for some people, to days or even weeks for others. The symptoms that accompany the head pain include nausea and vomiting, sensory sensitivity, body and mind fatigue, loss of some cognitive function, numbness, eye and neck

3

pain, and so many more. The literary works that describe this phase, including Marilyn Hacker's "Headaches" and Iman Mersal's "I Describe a Migraine" are charged with fierceness—warlike, violent imagery and fragmented lines and line breaks, capturing the utter chaos sufferers feel in their brains and body:

> Tortured syntax, thorned thoughts, vocabulary
> like a forest littered with unexploded
> cluster bombs, no exit except explosion
> ripping the branches.[2]

The final works in this part take us into the last phase, the Postdrome Phase. After the piercing headache has lifted, at least somewhat, most migraineurs commonly experience what feels like a "hangover." Again, the symptoms and longevity of this last stage vary significantly, though many share the "migraine fog," a heaviness, and exhaustion. For those with chronic migraine, the cycle moves in and out of and back and forth among these phases; the cycle seems to go on and on, with the migraine event rarely fully lifting. Looking as far back as medieval poet William Dunbar's "On His Heid-ake" we see the symptoms we well recognize: "Though I tried to start writing, / The sense was difficult to find, / Deep down sleepless in my head, / Dulled in dullness and distress."[3]

The writers in this part have taken the experience of migraine and transferred it to a medium that allows the sufferer and the nonsufferer to connect more meaningfully. If you are reading "What It Feels Like" as a family member of one who suffers from a migraine—spouse, partner, sibling, parent, or child—you will find in these selections a way to help you read differently and more accurately the person in your life. For example, Paula Kamen, in her essay "Down the Rabbit Hole," describes how, in addition to the many triggers of migraine, stress is a major trigger, though our culture expects that someone experiencing stress will be able "with the proper discipline" to control that emotion: "The pain is easily triggered by external and internal forces, such as stress, which are often mistakenly labeled the root cause. All this confusion is further compounded by the multiple forms that migraine takes, all theoretically originating from one basic problem: *a neurological dysfunction in the brain stem*."[4] After reading her essay, you may be more compassionate, knowing that it's not the emotional outburst that is caused by a lack of moral discipline or control but rather the deep disease that often masks itself under more familiar behavior.

As a person close to the sufferer, you may develop acumen for detecting patterns of triggers and warning signs, some of which the migraineur herself may not yet recognize. For example, as Jean Hanson notes in her essay "The Lightning in My Eyes," often it's a husband who notices the early symptoms before you do: "a certain posture in your sleep and a slowness in your reasoning," or, as she also explains, "Your sister hears it in your legato voice: There's not melody, she says, you've gone flat."[5]

Practitioners (headache specialists, general neurologists, primary care physicians, and students studying medicine) will benefit from reading about the widespread, not always immediate, symptoms of migraine that run throughout the works in this part. Gaining these insights might lead them to more compassion and directed questions for patients; they might encourage them to create a physical environment more conducive to the needs of migraine sufferers. Laurie Batitto Bisconti's "The Patient's Perspective: A Friend Like No Other" shows, from a patient's point of view, the fierceness and constancy of chronic migraine. The fictional rendering of Nietzsche, in Irvin Yalom's "When Nietzsche Wept," records the astonishment of Dr. B. when he realizes for the first time, "such a situation—the majority of one's days are torment, a handful of healthy days a year, one's life consumed by pain."[6]

General readers will benefit from learning more about living with episodic and chronic illness. Often, people look at migraineurs differently and largely without understanding. The sufferer knows the public stares when she has trouble coming up with words, has difficulty putting a coherent sentence together, or is constantly pushing on a specific spot on the side of her neck. The loss of cognitive function, the fog that takes over, in stages other than the full-blown migraine, the hangover from the full-blown migraine—all of these additional symptoms are commonplace for the sufferer but appear to the outsider as strange and often alienate the sufferer from friends, colleagues, and the general public.

Anna Leahy's essay "Half-Skull Days," one of the two essays given prominence by beginning and ending the anthology, beautifully captures this stressful, anxiety-producing aspect of migraine for so many sufferers and those around them:

> The staved-off migraine's disorientation has left me aware of my own incoherence, my inability to track time accurately or to guess what I might say next, or not be able to say. When I couldn't think of the word *scale*, upon which I had slammed my toe and made a racket in the bathroom only moments before, I pantomimed stepping onto the scale and looking down to see my weight. But even my husband is not used to this sort of communication and shrugged; at least he was no longer worried that I'd injured myself. I would not call what I felt in this semi-articulate moment *pain*, but I was suffering.[7]

All audiences will benefit from learning and feeling the joy and subsequent fear the migraineur experiences when, after days, weeks, or months of being caught up in the migraine cycle, nearly forgetting what it's like to feel "good and normal," the cycle lifts, fully "breaks," and often brings the person with migraine a euphoric feeling that takes over her whole self:

What's not invisible is the ecstasy of waking up and knowing right away that the migraine cycle has broken; I lift my head on these days feeling like a real force has moved out of my brain and body; suddenly, I'm me again. Do some people wake up this way most days? I never have more gratitude and mindfulness than I do when I experience this "lift." I pay attention to all the beauty of the day, and I have energy because now I can live rather than exist—at least for this moment.[8]

These are the days both the migraineur and all of those close to her live for.

NOTES

1. Linda Pastan, "Migraine," in *An Early Afterlife* (New York: W. W. Norton, 1995), lines 1–4.
2. Marilyn Hacker, "Headaches," from *A Stranger's Mirror: New and Selected Poems: 1994–2014* (New York: W. W. Norton: 2015), lines 5–8.
3. William Dunbar, "On His Heid-ake," in *The Poems of William Dunbar*, ed. W. Mackay Mackenzie (London: Faber and Faber, 1932), lines 7–10.
4. Paula Kamen, "Down the Rabbit Hole," in *All in My Head* (Boston: Da Capo, 2005), 23.
5. Jean Hanson, "The Lightning in My Eyes," in *A View from the Divide: Creative Nonfiction on Health and Science* (Pittsburgh: Univ. of Pittsburgh Press, 1998), 43.
6. Irvin Yalom, *When Nietzsche Wept* (New York: Harper Perennial, 2003), 71.
7. Anna Leahy, "Half-Skull Days," *The Pinch* 32, no. 1 (2012): 244.
8. Kathleen J. O'Shea, "I Know Upon Awakening," in *So Much More Than a Headache: Understanding Migraine through Literature* (Kent, OH: Kent State Univ. Press, 2020), 141.

Warning Signs

Migraine

LINDA PASTAN

Ambushed by
pins and needles
of light . . . by jagged

voices . . . strobes . . .
the sanctuary is taken
from within.

I am betrayed by
the fractured
senses. I

crouch on the
tilting floor of
consciousness, fearing

the eggshell
skull won't hold,
will crack,

as the lid is tightened
another implacable
inch. I would

banish every
blessing—these
shooting

stars . . . the future . . .
all brilliant
excitations—just for

silence or sleep
or the cotton wool
of the perfected dark.

Patterns

OLIVER SACKS

I have had migraines for most of my life; the first attack I remember occurred when I was 3 or 4 years old. I was playing in the garden when a brilliant, shimmering light appeared to my left—dazzlingly bright, almost as bright as the sun. It expanded, becoming an enormous shimmering semicircle stretching from the ground to the sky, with sharp zigzagging borders and brilliant blue and orange colors. Then, behind the brightness, came a blindness, an emptiness in my field of vision, and soon I could see almost nothing on my left side. I was terrified—what was happening? My sight returned to normal in a few minutes, but these were the longest minutes I had ever experienced.

I told my mother what had happened, and she explained to me that what I had had was a migraine—she was a doctor, and she, too, was a migraineur. It was a "visual migraine," she said, or a migraine "aura." The zigzag shape, she would later tell me, resembled that of medieval forts, and was sometimes called a "fortification pattern." Many people, she explained, would get a terrible headache after seeing such a "fortification"—but, if I were lucky, I would be one of those who got only the aura, without the headache.

I was lucky here, and lucky, too, to have a mother who could reassure me that everything would be back to normal within a few minutes, and with whom, as I got older, I could share my migraine experiences. She explained that auras like mine were due to a sort of disturbance like a wave passing across the visual parts of the brain. A similar "wave" might pass over other parts of the brain, she said, so one might get a strange feeling on one side of the body, or experience a funny smell, or find oneself temporarily unable to speak. A migraine might affect one's perception of color, or depth, or movement, might make the whole visual world unintelligible for a few minutes. Then, if one were unlucky, the rest of the migraine might follow: violent headaches, often on one side, vomiting, painful sensitivity to light and noise, abdominal disturbances, and a host of other symptoms.

In her memoir, *Giving Up the Ghost,* the British novelist Hilary Mantel describes the migraines she started to have in early childhood:

My eyes are drawn to a spot. . . . I can't see anything, not exactly see: except the faintest movement, a ripple, a disturbance of the air. I can sense a spiral, a lazy buzzing swirl, like flies; but it is not flies. There is nothing to see. There is nothing to smell. There is nothing to hear. But its motion, its insolent shift, makes my stomach heave. I can sense—at the periphery, the limit of all my senses—the dimensions of the creature. It is as high as a child of two. Its depth is a foot, fifteen inches. . . . . It has no edges, no mass, no dimension, no shape except the formless; it moves. . . . . Within the space of a thought it is inside me, and has set up a sick resonance within my bones and in all the cavities of my body.

For Mantel, as a child, migraine "charged [the air] with invisible presences and the echoes of strangers' voices; it gave me morbid visions." She writes:

Sometimes the aura takes more trying forms. I will go deaf. The words I try to write end up as other words. I will suffer strange dreams, from which I wake with hallucinations of taste. . . . . A tune will lodge in my head like a tic, and bring the words tripping in with it. . . . It's a familiar complaint, to have tune you can't get out of your head. But for most people the tunes aren't the prelude to a day of hearty vomiting.

For a time, as a child, Mantel saw "a constant, moving backdrop of tiny skulls . . . skulls skulls skulls, the size of my little fingernail, unrolling . . . like a satanist's wallpaper."

Seeing multitudes of tiny, identical structures, sometimes "unrolling" steadily, sometimes flickering, forming and reforming, all over the visual field, is common in migraine auras, though it is only occasionally that these are elaborated into tiny skulls, or arrays of faces or animals or other objects.

In my own migraine auras, I would sometimes see—vividly with closed eyes, more faintly and transparently if I kept my eyes open—tiny branching lines, like twigs, or geometrical structures covering the entire visual field: lattices, checkerboards, cobwebs, and honeycombs. Sometimes there were more elaborate patterns, like Turkish carpets or complex mosaics; sometimes I saw scrolls and spirals, swirls and eddies; sometimes three-dimensional shapes like tiny pine cones or sea urchins.

Such patterns, I found, were not peculiar to me, and years later, when I worked in a migraine clinic, I discovered that many of my patients habitually saw such patterns. And when I looked back on historical accounts, I found that Sir John Herschel, the astronomer, had given detailed descriptions of his own visual migraines in the 1850s. He wrote to his fellow astronomer and fellow migraineur, George Airy, quoting his own notes: "The fortification pattern twice in my eyes today. . . . Also a sort of chequer work filling in, in rectangular patches, and a carpet-work pattern over the rest of the visual area." Herschel wondered whether there might be "a kaleidoscopic power in the sensorium to form regular patterns by the symmetrical combination of casual elements," a power "working within our own organization [but] distinct from that of our own personality."

Many years later, as a young doctor, I read a little book (really two little books) by the great neurologist Heinrich Klüver, "Mescal" and "Mechanisms of Hallucination." Klüver not only culled many accounts from the literature, but experimented with mescal himself, and described geometric visual hallucinations typical of the early stages of the mescal experience: "Transparent oriental rugs, but infinitely small . . . plastic filigreed spherical objets d'art [like] radiolaria . . . wallpaper designs . . . cobweb-like figures or concentric circles and squares . . . architectural forms, buttresses, rosettes, leafwork, fretwork."

Klüver spoke here of hallucinatory "form constants" and the tendency to "geometrization," to the "geometrical-ornamental," seemingly built into the brain-mind. The visions produced by mescal and other hallucinogens would usually progress from these elementary forms of hallucination to elaborate visions of a much more personal and sometimes mystical sort (including scenes of people, animals, and landscapes). But Klüver remarked that the lower-level, geometric hallucinations that preceded these were identical to those found in a variety of conditions: migraine, sensory deprivation, low blood sugar, fever, delirium, or the hypnopompic and hypnagogic states that come immediately before and after sleep. Indeed, even in the absence of any special medical conditions, they could be evoked in anyone by flickering lights, or sometimes even by simply applying pressure to the eyes.

Such geometrical form constants, then, are not dependent on memory or personal experience or desire or imagination. And for those of us with migraine auras—perhaps 10 percent of the population—they are almost like old friends.

Though migraine causes great suffering for millions of people, there has been much success, in the last decade or two, in understanding what goes on during attacks, and how to prevent or minimize them. But we still have only a very primitive understanding of what, to my mind, are among the most intriguing phenomena of migraine—the geometric hallucinations it so often evokes. What we can say, in general terms, is that these hallucinations reflect the minute anatomical organization, the cytoarchitecture, of the primary visual cortex, including its columnar structure—and the ways in which the activity of millions of nerve cells organizes itself to produce complex and ever-changing patterns. We can actually see, through such hallucinations, something of the dynamics of a large population of living nerve cells and, in particular, the role of what mathematicians term deterministic chaos in allowing complex patterns of activity to emerge throughout the visual cortex. This activity operates at a basic cellular level, far beneath the level of personal experience. They are archetypes, in a way, universals of human experience.

As a child, I was fascinated by patterns, starting with the patterns in our house—the square colored floor tiles we had on the porch, the tessellation of small pentagonal and hexagonal ones in the kitchen; the herringbone pattern on the curtains in my room, and the pattern on my father's check suit. When I was taken to the synagogue for services, I was more interested in the mosaics of tiny tiles on the floor than in the religious liturgy. And I was fascinated by a pair of antique Chinese cabinets we had in our drawing room, for embossed on their lacquered surfaces were patterns of wonderful intricacy, patterns on different scales, patterns nested within patterns, all surrounded by clusters of tendrils and leaves.

These geometric and scrolling motifs seemed somehow familiar to me, though it did not dawn on me until years later that this was because I had seen them not only in my environment but in my own head, that these patterns resonated with my own inner experience of the intricate tilings and swirls of migraine.

Much later still, when I first saw photographs of the Alhambra, with its intricate geometric mosaics, I started to wonder whether what I had taken to be a personal experience and resonance might in fact be part of a larger whole, whether certain basic forms of geometric art, going back for tens of thousands of years, might also reflect the external expression of universal experiences. Migraine-like patterns, so to speak, are seen not only in Islamic art, but in classical and medieval motifs, in Zapotec architecture, in the bark paintings of Aboriginal artists in Australia, in Acoma pottery, in Swazi basketry—in virtually every culture. There seems to have been, throughout human history, a need to externalize, to make art from, these internal experiences, from the decorative motifs of prehistoric cave paintings to the psychedelic art of the 1960s. Do the arabesques in our own minds, built into our own brain organization, provide us with our first intimations of geometry, of formal beauty?

Whether or not this is the case, there is an increasing feeling among neuro-scientists that self-organizing activity in vast populations of visual neurons is a prerequisite of visual perception—that this is how seeing begins. Spontaneous self-organization is not restricted to living systems—one may see it equally in the formation of snow crystals, in the roilings and eddies of turbulent water, in certain oscillating chemical reactions. Here, too, self-organization can produce geometries and patterns in space and time, very similar to what one may see in a migraine aura. In this sense, the geometrical hallucinations of migraine allow us to experience in ourselves not only a universal of neural functioning, but a universal of nature itself.

Down the Rabbit Hole

PAULA KAMEN

In the original Alice's *Adventures in Wonderland* and *Through the Looking-Glass* of the late nineteenth century (as well as in the Disney cartoon version, which I am more familiar with), the characters face many absurdities and illusions. Not the least of which is headache.

After reading the *Wonderland* book, no one would be surprised to learn that the author, Lewis Carroll, was a migraine sufferer. In one chapter, the Queen of Hearts complains of a "forehead ache," and in another Tweedledee comments, "Generally I am very brave . . . only today I happen to have a headache."

Yet, other parts of Alice's journey down the rabbit hole and through the looking glass—which do not specifically address this ailment—also serve well to illustrate the generally confusing and topsy-turvy nature of the chronic headache experience.

Likewise, the world of headache treatment is one of doublespeak and doubt: a world where decisions made by the authorities around you seem arbitrary, where you suddenly find yourself on trial when no crime has been committed, where sentences (or courses of action) are decided well before any sound verdicts or diagnoses are handed down, where one mysterious potion begging, "Drink me," unexpectedly turns your life upside down, and where, worst of all, you cannot trust the logic of your own senses to guide you through it all.

"Alice felt dreadfully puzzled," Carroll wrote, describing her reaction to the Mad Hatter at the tea party, a comment that could, in my view, describe a patient's state of mind after a typically brief conversation with a high-level medical specialist: "The Hatter's remark seemed to her to have no sort of meaning in it, and yet it was certainly English."

Indeed, the world of chronic pain and headache is essentially one of illusion. Here, not only does one appear crazy but also commonly privately wonders if he or she has reached that point.

In fact, as I learned only years later, the migraine experience, which takes on endless types of forms and symptoms, is often hard-wired for such a seemingly crazy trip.

This "trippy-ness" may characterize all stages of the attack. Before the pain sets in, many patients experience a variety of bizarre neurological events, which doctors actually refer to as the *Alice in Wonderland* phenomenon, and which at first may seem like hints of a nervous breakdown. About 20–70 percent of migraine patients have *prodrome,* or *premonitory phenomena,* hours and even days before the migraine attack. A prodrome may include extremes of elation or depression, strong food cravings, and insomnia.

Then, when the migraine phase hits, distortions may intensify. Besides the terrible pain, complaints may include oversensitivity to light, sounds, and smells; difficulty in integrating mental activities, such as speaking or reading or writing; nausea and vomiting; feelings of fear and delirium; numbness in the extremities; widespread pain; and a sense of being detached from one's surroundings. For this reason, migraine has historically been labeled *sick headache:* General Ulysses S. Grant famously reported suffering one before Lee surrendered to him in the Civil War.

Some of Alice's most seemingly idiosyncratic adventures illustrate other very specific neurological effects. The patient may feel too big for his or her surroundings, as in Alice's experience of almost bursting a small cottage after drinking one of her tonics. She also describes tunnel vision and vertigo, which migraine sufferers may also experience.

For about 20–60 percent of migraine sufferers, a visual aura appears in the hour before the pain descends. (This type of headache is now, rather plainly, classified as *migraine with aura* and was formerly called *classic migraine.* It contrasts to *migraine without aura,* formerly called *common migraine.*) This aura, which either disappears with the onset of the pain or accompanies it, typically goes on for less than an hour, but it sometimes reappears for days.

In about 20 percent of these cases of aura, no pain follows the aura at all. This aura experience without pain mainly happens to children and also describes twilight states involved in other neurological problems, such as epilepsy, Epstein-Barr virus, and schizophrenia. In fact, this aura trip strongly resembles what one would see with certain hallucinogens, such as LSD and those funny little mushrooms. This aura all happens within the brain, as a result of brainwave changes. The phenomenon does not result from changes taking place in the eyes themselves. And this light show varies greatly from person to person, and even from attack to attack. During an aura, the internal brain can broadcast to itself a festival of twinkling stars, called *phosphenes.* Some shapes are bigger blobs called *scotomas*—also referred to as *negative scotomas*—which may actually act as blind spots and blot out what you see before you, the effect being like that of a hole in a movie screen. Patients have reported their visual fields broken up by honeycomb patterns, bizarre tiltings, and cubistlike mosaic visions—the type of special effects that you would expect to see in a psychedelic 1960s video with The Doors music in the background.

Some auras feature particular types of zigzag shapes, called *fortifications*. A term also used is *teichopsia,* which is Greek for "town wall" and "vision." In reality, these shapes really do resemble, from an aerial view, the protective, fortifying battlements around medieval towns. (Driving home this point, the migraine textbook, *Headache in Clinical Practice,* actually gives a photo of the walled city of Palmanova, Italy, to illustrate a "migraine with aura." To use a more modern metaphor, these structures resemble a ring or horseshoe made of Legos, or an aerial view of an urban mid-twentieth-century courtyard apartment building, the kind that my grandmother lived in.)

Although typical episodic migraine attacks of all types may last less than a day, often under two hours, some may go on for days and/or occur many times a week, blurring the line with, and even evolving into, chronic daily headache. Afterward, as is typical of drug trips, some patients feel refreshed and euphoric, and others are depressed and fatigued.

In my particular case, at the beginning of 1999, after my surgery, I felt as if I had been under the spell of other types of illusions. I was troubled, especially because of my personal complicity in this surgery, by how strong my powers of self-delusion could be. Again, I had seen what I had wanted to see. I realized that when I was dealing with pain, even the "concrete" was really not concrete. This nasal obstruction of the septum that I could feel and see (with a brain scan), which physically dug right into the site of pain behind my eye, was just a red herring. I was as confused as Alice at the tea party.

Finally, about a month and a half after the surgery, the blood in my eye slowly faded away. The intense broken-glass feeling in the left eye subsided, and I happily stopped taking those fog-inducing Lortabs and Lorcets. I was left with a headache slightly worse than the one I had started out with. What was also distressing, I was even more confused about the source of the pain. I had followed a trail of seemingly stunning clues that all turned out to be dead ends.

Like many patients, I was still having trouble distinguishing common *symptoms* of migraine (such as neck pain and allergy) from the original causes. I also was confused by how structural abnormalities (like a deviated septum) might not necessarily cause the pain. "Indeed," commented Oliver Sacks, in his book *Migraine,* "there is probably no field in medicine so strewn with the debris of misdiagnosis and mistreatment, and of well-intentioned but wholly mistaken medical and surgical intervention."

After recognizing how strongly external stimuli triggered the pain, as the surgery had ignited it to kingdom come, I continued to wonder about recent diagnoses, for example, if this condition was really neuralgia. To get an answer, I saw a prominent pain specialist, one whom my mother happened to spot on the cover of *Chicago Magazine,* who was billed as one of the best doctors in the city. I considered myself lucky to get an appointment. Telling me that my pain was too constant to qualify as neuralgia, he presented another seemingly rational question: Was it from stenosis?

After giving me some MRIs of the neck and brain, the only irregularity he found was a mild stenosis (a spinal narrowing) at the base of the neck. As a treatment, he wanted to do a "bilateral facet nerve block" injection of an anesthetic into the spinal cord at the point of the stenosis. This was a diagnostic tool. If the injection got rid of the pain, the stenosis was the source of the problem and I could have some radiofrequency work done to more permanently sever the nerve at that point. But I declined. I didn't have the stamina to undergo any more invasive procedures involving doctors wielding large and sharp objects near my head and spine—no matter how stellar their qualifications seemed. And my uncle, along with other doctors I would see later, said that stenosis that low in the spine would lead to shoulder or arm pain, not headache pain. My uncle observed that most people have some irregularities in the spine, but they are not all a source of pain. Still, I felt wracked with doubt that I was leaving a major clue unexplored.

At that time, I did not know the basic medical information that I now have—about why so many false clues exist, and about why chronic headache is so prone to misdiagnosis and needless and even harmful procedures. Once again, as with the widespread confusion about headaches as psychosomatic, its inherently invisible *neurological basis* is the culprit. The pain is easily triggered by external and internal forces, such as stress, which are often mistakenly labeled the root cause. All this confusion is further compounded by the multiple forms that migraine takes, all theoretically originating from one basic problem: *a neurological dysfunction in the brain stem.*

As Dr. Scott Fishman wrote in his insightful book *The War on Pain,* a point of origin of all these seeming illusions is thought to be the thalamus, the command center of the brain for controlling pain and emotion. In some people who are genetically predisposed, the thalamus overinterprets even the most minor triggers, internal and external—hormones, the weather, stress, chemicals in food, and so on. When stimulated, the thalamus sends a cascade of signals throughout the brain. Some of these are neurological and are associated with classic migraine, such as nausea; loss of appetite; oversensitivity to light, sound, and smell; visual aura; and numbness in the body.

In addition, this cascade of activity sparked by the thalamus may create muscle tension in the neck and shoulders, which is often mistaken for the root cause of headache pain—as I had experienced with physical therapy and massage therapists. Along with these processes, blood vessels on the periphery of the brain expanded can also trigger sinus pain.

In reality, as many patients and doctors never realize, these sinus problems can be a *result* of the migraine's neurological chain of events, not a cause of it. Specifically, this reaction irritates the trigeminal nerve, which supplies sensation to the face and head. The long trigeminal nerve has branches that also go into the sinuses and the nasal cavities. This process may also stimulate sinus problems, which accompany an estimated 45 percent of migraine attacks. A recent study revealed that nine out of ten patients who had been diagnosed with sinus headaches really had migraines.

The connection between the inflamed trigeminal nerve and sinus symptoms also explains the connection between migraine and sinus medications. Migraine sufferers have found that triptans, such as Imitrex, can relieve their sinus problems. Many of us have also found that inflammation-shrinking decongestants, such as the Tavist D that I have relied on, can help relieve headache pain. A resulting and often false assumption is that if sinus medication helps the headache, the headache is based in sinus problems.

Another major mix-up in treating chronic headache is in blaming stress as the root cause of chronic pain, instead of a trigger.

In truth, a person has to have a genetic predisposition to chronic headaches to have them. After all, saying stress causes a headache is like saying cold weather causes a flu or a smoky room causes asthma. A person has these vulnerabilities to begin with. As Susan Sontag wrote in *Illness as Metaphor:* "Needless to say, the hypothesis that distress can affect immunological responsiveness (and, in some circumstances, lower immunity to disease) is hardly the same as—or constitutes evidence for—the view that emotions cause diseases, much less for the belief that specific emotions can produce specific diseases."

This distinction can be more confusing for those patients for whom stress is the major trigger. Stress is more morally charged than other triggers, such as certain foods and weather changes. Stress is less "legitimate" because it involves emotions, which anyone with proper discipline is expected to control. And so, this factor of emotion—equated for decades with "hysteria"—becomes the most visible culprit, *rather than* a person's neurobiological predisposition.

In fact, confusion also arises because stress is the most commonly reported trigger for all types of headaches, between one-third and two-thirds of patients reporting it as an influence. It invariably rates high on the list, even above foods and hormones. But many people have chronic headaches with no identifiable triggers, either internal or external. And stress is also a factor in every other illness. Stress can worsen, merely accompany, or result from diabetes, cancer, hypertension, Parkinson's disease, and so on.

Not that trying to reduce and manage stress is a bad idea. Reducing stress's impact as a trigger may also raise the threshold for getting a headache (or a worse headache, for those who have it constantly). In most people, triggers are considered "additive," each one making a difference only when many pile up. These triggers all work together to raise a person's vulnerability to the migraine attack. I've heard this dynamic described as each trigger contributing to lighting a part of the fuse, which varies in length among individuals. (And people with chronic headaches have unusually short fuses.) In other words, a person may not get a headache from lack of sleep, hormone fluctuation, or Parmesan cheese, but when all are experienced at once, the opportunistic pain breaks through.

In reality, another reason why stress is *not* the root cause of chronic pain, although it is definitely a trigger, is that stress is a fact of life for just about everyone. It's true that we can learn to manage it better, but it's hard to stop major and minor stressful events from happening in the first place, while we are still trying to live in the real world—and not in some kind of plastic bubble. Blaming pain on stress could be compared to blaming hormones for causing a woman's depression. Every woman of reproductive age has fluctuating hormones, but not every woman gets depressed as a result. The more fundamental culprit is individual brain chemistry, which determines a woman's neurological response to hormones, not the hormones themselves.

One neurologist I interviewed in 2003, Dr. Vincent Martin, also a headache sufferer, explained the concept of triggers to me in another way, by calling an overly sensitive nervous system the main problem: "So you've got this nervous system that's overreactive to both your internal and your external environment. So all these triggers are floating around out there. Internally, there are the hormonal changes. Then another trigger would be stress. The more stress you have, the more headaches you get. You might eat the wrong foods; you might drink too much coffee and develop caffeine-withdrawal headaches. Weather changes might bother you. So it's as if in this particular nervous system every change in the environment actually provokes a headache. And that's a system that you live with and I live with, and it's just a very sensitive type of nervous system.

"So everything provokes a headache. I have heard that so often from chronic daily headache patients: 'Dr. Martin, everything provokes a headache. I mean, if I eat, if I sleep too much or sleep too little, if I get, you know, get a little distressed, if I have a beer . . . ' And they just feel frustrated because they feel that everything they potentially do or all the good things in life are going to provoke a headache."

As with other types of confusion, the media have played a large part in this widespread misunderstanding of the role of triggers, by not reporting the distinctions. You can just skim the headlines of major stories about chronic headaches to get the drift. A story in the July 14, 2003, *Los Angeles Times* explained why "That Raging Headache May be Anger Based." It reported research from St. Louis University finding that headache sufferers are more likely to hold in anger. That may be true, but the article does not explain that this anger is a trigger, not a root cause. An article in the February 2004 issue of *Redbook* informs you "Why You've Got That Headache," listing six surprising causes, which range from holding in anger to changing sleeping patterns on the weekends. Although the article itself refers to these provocations as "triggers," it does not talk about a genetic predisposition to having headaches in the first place. Although helpful, because they encourage good anger and stress management, reports such as these also compound the guilt that headache sufferers feel because they suspect they are essentially bringing headaches on themselves and are emotionally disturbed.

Furthermore, this complex and invisible neurological process leads to another source of confusion, a misdiagnosis of the *type* of headache suffered. Is it migraine, tension headache, chronic daily headache, or trigeminal neuralgia, I have asked myself at different times, while in pursuit of different courses of treatment. But as some doctors now theorize, these may all be different manifestations of the *same* problem, a basic stimuli-processing dysfunction in the thalamus.

Compounding problems is many pain practitioners' lack of understanding of these neurological processes. As a result, practitioners see what they want to see, the headache functioning as one big inkblot test (or as Charlie from *Flowers for Algnernon* would say, "*ror shak* test"). Massage therapists see muscle tension as the root of headaches; ENT specialists diagnose sinus problems; and chiropractors blame spinal deformities. Some of this prejudice is human nature. Indeed, "when the only tool you own is a hammer, every problem begins to resemble a nail" goes the famous quote from Abraham Maslow. (A friend's retina-surgeon husband cited this to me after my surgery.)

Even so, paying attention to the symptoms of chronic headache is important. Addressing them can be a step toward at least raising the body's resistance to pain. Just like treating sinus problems, treating the muscle pain resulting from a migraine may, at least temporarily, help relieve the headache. The challenge is to attack the headache at any point along the chain of events from the thalamus (with antiepileptic drugs) to trigger points on the shoulders (with massage). I have heard of some people getting relief with a dental guard at night that prevents them from clenching their jaw, which could contribute to exacerbating the pain (but may not necessarily be the root cause).

Symptom chasing should be done realistically and responsibly. At best, relieving these problems might reduce headache pain, raising one's resistance to headaches in the first place. But at worst, aggressively treating what turns out to be a false lead, as in the case of my surgery, can make the pain worse.

Unfortunately, as I found out only recently, I was not alone in having surgery for no reason—for confusing a symptom (sinus problems) with the cause. In his

2002 guide *Heal Your Headache*, Dr. David Buchholz reported that surgeries on the sinuses and other structural areas of the head, such as a deviated septum "pressing against something," are common among chronic headache patients. He even profiled one patient who had six such surgeries before seeing him. He added that he has personally treated six women who had previously had breast reduction surgery to cure their migraines, in an effort to reduce stress on nerves, such as from bra straps straining the shoulders. These surgeries also failed.

Surgical efforts to relieve pain are notoriously risky and generally ineffective. Doctors through history have discovered this after severing irritated nerves, only to see the pain return in another part of the body, and more severely. Much of the programming of pain is seated in the thalamus, and no matter which nerves are severed in the body, the aberrant signals from the thalamus persist. As in my case, brain scans fail to show the definitive source of pain and are all open to interpretation. Even a structural irregularity, such as a deviated septum or a stenosis of the spinal cord, may be red herrings, typical even in people who have no pain.

I discovered another disturbing risk while attending the annual meeting of the American Pain Society in March 2003: Many invasive procedures have not been adequately tested. "Proper research is rarely undertaken and typically comes late, often 10 to 20 years after the first invention of the procedure," said Dr. Nikolai Bogduk, a prominent Australian pain researcher and authority on evidence-based medicine (or that tiny part of medicine that has been scientifically "proven"). "This is opposite to the way scientists behave in other disciplines, where if the results are negative, that should lead to cessation of the procedure. This never happens. Once it's established, despite the evidence, invasive procedures keep being perpetuated."

Dr. Bogduk warned that doctors often skip important precautionary steps for the sake of convenience, even with procedures that have been proven to work. (In my case, the ENT surgeon didn't give me any kind of control nerve block near the deviated septum, to confirm that this was the culprit.) This failure commonly occurs with nerve blocks themselves, used to relieve pain. Dr. Bogduk said that giving the patient a saline (saltwater) block in addition to one with real anesthesia can easily demonstrate if the procedure has a placebo effect. This precaution can reduce the expense and danger of follow-up surgery to actually sever the suspected nerve.

At that same conference, in a major speech to the hundreds assembled, Dr. John D. Loeser warned that the same problem in using "off-label" drugs exists with "off-label" surgery. A procedure, such as a type of nerve block, may be approved by the FDA for one problem but not for a host of others, for which it eventually may become routine. He said that doctors too often resort to such "quick fixes" instead of spending the time to get to know the patient and treat pain in other ways. "It is not that I am opposed to interventions, for I earn my living as a neurosurgeon," he said. "I do recognize, however, that every needle has a sharp end that goes into the patient and a blunt end that is attached to a provider. And every scalpel has a blade that encroaches upon the patient and a handle that attaches to a surgeon. Anyone who thinks that all the action occurs at the sharp end does not understand either health care or human behavior."

But doctors tend to communicate poorly with patients about the complexities of surgery. Needless to say, the media further contribute to this poor understanding and may unrealistically fan the hopes of patients. As when promoting "wonder drugs," the media often follow a formula that points to technology as a "quick fix." Features often focus on those who are helped but neglect to cover those who aren't. Or they might ignore possible major and likely side effects.

A flaw in statistics adds confusion. Negative results of off-label uses are rarely or never, and positive results (fudged or not) are always, published. Out of 1,000 studies, by chance 50 will show significant improvement at the 95 percent confidence level, leading the talking heads on 10 P. M. newscasts to proclaim, "New hope for sufferers." The other 950 studies will never appear on a printed page or on the air.

On one level, of course, journalistic coverage of surgical alternatives can be helpful, to give patients more options to consider and bring up with their doctors. But the typically narrow and totally uncritical coverage often does more of a disservice in the long run, as it lacks a realistic assessment of the complexities and risks of such surgery. The news peg is that the surgery worked for this one person here and therefore can work for *you*. But the stories fail to convey the bigger picture.

Another motivation contributing to pursuit of the hazard-strewn path of surgery for chronic pain is more craven: financial.

Invasive procedures and surgeries are a major method of making money from headache patients. Some of this work can be done in less than an hour and earn the practitioner thousands of dollars, with the endorsement of insurance companies, which trust surgery to be a "real" treatment. In contrast, the other ways that doctors treat pain, through getting to know the patient, are not so remunerative.

Typically, a neurologist or internist will see a pain patient infrequently, for a relatively small office-visit fee (such as seventy-five to a hundred dollars), and then that patient will eat up her or his time with phone calls about medications and changing symptoms. As an example of the time required to treat such patients, in his textbook for doctors about pain medications, *Management of Headache and Headache Medications,* Dr. Lawrence Robbins outlines typical case studies that require dozens of phone calls back and forth. One example is given in his two-plus-page (small-type) summary of his months-long treatment of Sally, a forty-five-year-old woman with "frequent migraine plus severe Chronic Daily Headache and menstrual migraine." After her initial office visit, her treatment involved constant phone calls to adjust the dosages and types of her three kinds of medication, abortive (to stem a migraine at its beginning), preventive (to take daily to increase her pain threshold), and palliative (just to ease the pain). He also noted her other health limits (e.g., a stomach that couldn't tolerate many anti-inflammatory drugs), the influence of comorbidities (insomnia, depression, anxiety), and the constantly changing side effects. By the end of the case study, Sally's headaches were better, but she was still working to balance side effects and relief. Despite all these months of work, her case remained a work in progress. Needless to say, paying such attention to the patient—necessary for adequate headache care with medications—is not the ideal way to drive up revenue. In contrast, a surgeon could cut into Sally's head and—in one hour—make a hundred times more profit. In that case, he or she would hardly have to bother to talk to Sally. The choices for many doctors, therefore, become very clear, whereas the patient continues to operate under the delusion that her best interests are being kept in mind—and that at long last, the medical world is about to come to its senses.

The Almanac Branch

BRADFORD MORROW

My migraines, which were alluded to as seldom as possible in our family, as if they were leprosy or madness, were referred to by us with the amiable old name of "megrim"—which sounded to me like "my grim," an accurate-enough homonym. They were the source, it was agreed by the several doctors to whom I'd been taken, of my visions . . . psychotic ecstasies, as one of the specialists—whom Faw loathed—called them; auras was Dr. Trudeau's word. Everyone was always more upset, and perhaps awed by the sheer phenomenological peculiarity of the visions than I, and as a result tended to ignore the migraine itself. For me, the auras, the whispering lights and fantastical occurrences, were indeed enthralling and even ecstatic, whereas the megrims that led to them were just weighty and deadening. During the megrims all I wanted was for my senses to stop receiving signals from the world, and for everything to come to an end. The megrims backed me into a dark wet quiet which, unlike the darkness my jolly haunted ailanthus tree thrived in, forbade growth. It is common for us to speak of St. Hildegard's sublime visions, when we speak of such things, and to marvel at her mystical stars and her descriptions of the city of God and the Fall of the Angels and all that stuff, but seldom do we think of her as just a pitiful girl racked by pains she didn't understand, and which to this day medicine has neither explained nor been able to cure. Rarely have I rued the fact we weren't religious. But when I have, I've fantasized what my so-called visions might have meant to me if we were. I could have been a saint, instead of Grace Brush. But some of the things I've done in life as a result of not believing I wouldn't give up for anything, let alone a martyr's seat up in big bad boring heaven. Let others retire in celestial peace and walk the Elysian Fields—which I picture as being a kind of golf course, pristine and manicured, with paths of raked stardust. For myself, give me my earthly weeds and I'll go my own direction. . . .

I didn't like, and still don't, people feeling sorry for me, so as often as not I did my best to mask what was going on. The flare man I can see in my mind's eye as clearly as if it had been yesterday, rather than a quarter of a century ago. If I hadn't lived in a migrainous world would I remember more about—and thus be able to better record—what our family was like before we left for the island? I'd like to think that I would have sharper memories of my brother Desmond. As it is, I do not. . . .

The Woman Lit by Fireflies

JIM HARRISON

SHE HAD NOT yet accepted as real the quiver in her stomach and the slight green dot of pain in the middle of her head that signaled an incipient migraine. Her husband on the car seat beside her punched in a tape called *Tracking the Blues* which contained no black music, but rather the witless drone of a weekly financial lecture sent from New York City. This particular tape was seven days stale and had been played three times on their trip, but Donald repeated it to get "fair value" for his money. The tape, not incidentally, replaced Stravinsky's *Histoire du Soldat* from an Iowa City FM station, a piece she always enjoyed.

"Do you mind, darling?" he asked.

"Not at all, dear," she replied, partly because the pain clinic she had attended in Arizona that spring had emphasized giving up resistance to outside phenomena at the possible onset of a migraine under the notion you wanted to starve rather than feed the affliction. For instance, she shouldn't have been driving—sitting with her eyes closed listening to music would have been helpful, but she drove to avoid reading to him, which is what he required when he drove. An additional, insurmountable problem was that his car, an Audi 5000, was low-slung and the early August corn beside Interstate 80 in Iowa presented itself as a dense green wall. She preferred the higher vantage of her own nine-year-old Toyota Land Cruiser, a functional clumsy old machine that she and her beloved friend Zilpha used on their outings, or so they called them, which were somewhat famous in their neighborhood in Bloomfield Hills, a suburb of Detroit.

Clare would be fifty in another week, Donald was fifty-one and eager to get on with life, a matter about which she had mixed feelings. They had just been visiting their daughter Laurel, who at twenty-nine was a veterinarian married to a veterinarian, the both of them ministering to horses and cattle in a clinic outside of Sioux City, Iowa, up near the Nebraska border. The visit had been cut short two days by a quarrel between Laurel and Donald. On the way home they were to spend the weekend with Donald Jr., who at twenty-seven was a commodities market whiz in Chicago.

"I love you, Mom, but I can't understand why you don't leave that asshole," Laurel had said.

"Please, Laurel, he's your father."

"In name only," she had replied, and then they kissed goodbye as they always did, with Clare's heart giving a breathless wrench at separation.

A specific giddiness began to overtake her when she thought of the goodbye. *This is the way, after all. I've spent my life,* she thought. You could not fault Donald for being Donald, any more than you could fault Laurel for being the same as she was at three years, a cantankerous little girl with a sure though general sense of mission, a personality so specific as to be sometimes offensive.

"The overloaded leverages are coming home to roost," Donald brayed so loud she applied the brakes. She quickly reset the cruise control at a modest seventy considering that most cars passed her at that speed. The week before at the club she attempted a witticism about how all the lives saved by the Mothers Against Drunk Driving were being lost to the raising of the speed limit. The luncheon ladies were used to Clare and let the quip pass, but not a new member who found it "dreadfully morbid." Suddenly it occurred to her that Donald didn't feel really good about making money unless others were losing theirs, which made it all, to her mind, a silly game to spend your life on rather than the grave process with which he was totally obsessed.

An ever so slight tremor of head pain made her dismiss the thought about Donald and money as true but banal. She forced her thoughts back to a pleasant morning with Laurel, spent hiking on some bluffs above the Missouri River. Laurel had discovered a rattlesnake that had difficulty getting out of their way because of a huge lump in its belly—no doubt, Laurel said, from swallowing a gopher. They both laughed when Laurel added, "Poor thing, also poor gopher." The laughter was nervous relief. The first hour of their walk had been spent lifting Clare's confusion over a pamphlet an anti-vivisectionist neighbor had given her concerning a doctor down south who, on a defense contract, had shot several thousand cats in the head for research. Laurel habitually defended the scientific community but this one puzzled her, as the brain of a cat was dissimilar enough to that of a human as to make the research appear useless. She did not tell Clare that it would have made more sense to shoot several thousand dogs, or better yet chimpanzees, though the latter were very expensive. The purpose of the research, of course, was to better treat head wounds in soldiers. . . .

At the time she could not believe [Donald's] brusque affability translated so well. They had dined nearly every evening with Italians he had met in his tours of brokerage offices, several times in their homes, allowing Clare a look into the life of Florence never allowed the ordinary tourist. Donald waved at her with the other hand on the phone, antsy to make his daily call. She watched him dial, then walked toward the Iowa Welcome Center and the adjoining bathrooms, her head beginning to thrum in the noisy heat. It occurred to her that the tourists all looked blowzy and fatigued because they were headed back east at the end of their vacations.

When she thought about it later Clare was surprised again by how clear and cool her painful mind had felt. Every human and object, the landscape itself, had the distinct outlines found in a coloring book before the crayons are applied. The green wall of the cornfield behind the Welcome Center became luminous and of surpassing loveliness. She turned and walked back toward Donald in the car but he was in his brokerage trance, his clipped business voice saying, "But what the hell happened to Isomet?"

In the bathroom stall she checked her bag for certain items: Donald Jr.'s Boy Scout compass she used on hikes with Zilpha, a small can of cranberry juice, the addresses of three orphan children she wrote to and helped support in Santo Domingo, Mexico and Costa Rica; in a leather packet was her passport and a copy of the new translation of the *Tao Te Ching* given to her by a counselor at the pain clinic, and at the bottom, and most important, was the tan beret she had bought thirty years before on Rue St.-Jacques and had never worn. As a comparative literature senior at Michigan State she was to spend a year studying in Paris which lasted only three weeks when her father died and the family sent her boyfriend Donald to fetch her home. At the time Donald wore lumberjack shirts, the only son in a working-class family from Flint, who intended to be a writer or labor leader. On dates they read John Dos Passo's *U. S. A.* trilogy aloud to each other. Curiously her father had rather liked Donald, and perhaps this was foresight into the man Donald would become. So each morning for three weeks in her tiny *pension* Clare would look at her beret but was too timid to put it on.

Now in the toilet stall she finally put on the beret and laughed softly to herself. It was so easy. For luck she also slipped on a conch pearl ring Zilpha had given her in March as a remembrance. Among her last words had been "We never got around to the Amazon," a trip they had planned since they were girls when they were convinced they'd discover a pleasanter civilization somewhere in the jungle. Clare took out a Cafergot pill, then put it back, preferring pain-ridden consciousness. She tried to remember something René Char had written, "Blank blank blank the legitimate fruits of daring," but the growing pain blinded her memory. The note itself was simple enough: "I am in a small red car driving east. My husband has been abusing me. Do not believe anything he says. Call my daughter." She added Laurel's number, wrote "To The Police" on the envelope and stuck it to the side of the stall with a postage stamp. She noted that someone had scratched "Bob is cute" with a sharp object on the paint and she smiled with the confusion of female and male.

Behind the Welcome Center a small boy walking the family dog held Clare's bag as she climbed the fence which was more difficult than she anticipated. She wobbled and the wire cut into the soles of her tennis shoes. On the other side she lost a few moments explaining to the boy why he couldn't go along, but then the dog started barking and she hurried off down between two corn rows, toward the interior, wherever that might be.

Within a scant five minutes Clare would have liked to turn around, had turning around not already become so improbable. A hundred yards into the cornfield the beret made her feel silly so she took it off and stuffed it into her bag. The moment the hat came off the pain became so excruciating she fell to her hands and knees and retched up her lunch of iced tea and a club sandwich. The pain was such that she could not balance herself on her hands and knees, but pushed her legs backward until she lay on her stomach. She closed her eyes a moment but the world became bright red and whirling. There was the slightest memory of a pain lesson but it was too abstract to be of much use: the secret was to maintain your equilibrium in the face of incomprehension, as pain, finally, could not be understood. . . .

Sun and Migraine

MURIEL NELSON

The blinds were up. I would have had them down
if they could keep light's blades outside. My view

was skewed, it's true or skewered—the right half to a
microscopic sea of ghosting cell shapes,

the left, to a distant sun it didn't want.
Emily Dickinson's funeral tramped through my brain

And split it with Auden's night that needs our love.
I turned the other cheek. One eye, pillowed

at a slant to the window, opened—an experiment—
the other, too, and then both halves together came

to be a black-shrouded firmament over waves
of quaking orange leaves and their shades. Brilliant

alders which had been looking sickly were losing
their grip when a seagull rose from them. Sparks

trailed, then feathers gathered and spread, speeding
from light into dark, and wings whitened, then blackened in
Flame.

The Lightning in My Eyes

JEAN HANSON

We're driving through South Dakota when I see the tall grass on the side of the road turn liquid. Then the plains come alive: They breathe and relax, breathe and relax. We could be in a boat on a golden ocean for all the dipping and swaying. After a while, the horizon flickers and sends up a filmy light. The air itself is viscous, moved by wind, distorting the landscape.

I close my eyes. It's been hot, an uncomfortable day for a long drive. We're going to visit my grandparents in the tiny town of Wilmot. I know this, of course, and yet at moments I feel I've left it behind and I'm observing myself, Jean, as if she is some curious artifact. When I open my eyes, flashes of lightning bolt across the sunny road. My husband Chris doesn't slow the car. The lightning is in my eyes, not in the atmosphere.

My grandmother, a woman with a face wrinkled like a dried peach, walks down the painted cement steps to greet us. We sit in the kitchen, and when I talk, my voice comes from the other side of the room, as if I am a ventriloquist. I press my index finger to my thumb, but my digits move through each other like gelatin, tingling. I am of the world, but I'm not.

My grandfather is thrilled with Chris, whom he keeps calling Pete. He displays the wooden coat hangers he carves, the best hangers in the world; he shows off his immaculate Buick, the best car in the world; he serves us Riunite, the best red wine—no, in honor of Pete, my husband of Sicilian heritage—the best *Italian* red wine in the world. I hear this as pleasing but insignificant background static.

Dinner is circular. Voices: first Jean's, then Chris's, Grandma's, Grandpa's, Jean, Chris. Serving dishes passed around and around the table. Forks moving in slow rotations around our plates. These spherical rituals are an orchestral accompaniment, my consciousness the melodic line moving above it. I am disengaged and hovering, monitoring Jean and the others. Chris puts his hand on my arm, as if to ground my flight, but I resist: I'm rising. My head is helium. I'm taking everything in, seeing patterns and meaning. I'm on the verge of understanding the whole, crazy, profound lot of it.

Only later is there nausea. In the guest room, I crawl into the bed my father was born in. He has died two months before. His high school graduation picture is on the bureau, and he watches as I leave his realm, the spirit world, and move into pain as pure as frozen winter, an icicle poked in my forehead.

If I ask you to define *migraine,* you will call it an excruciating headache. Well, yes. And no. For those like me—among the distinct minority who suffer "classic" (with aura) rather than "common" migraine—the journey is more circuitous.

On days when you're singing through the mundane details of life, admiring the warmest chambers of your husband's heart and feeling lucky, you may be on the verge of a migraine. The migraine precursor is often a nearly euphoric sense of well-being—George Eliot described it as feeling "dangerously well." It can also manifest as apprehension, a texture of strangeness. You can't shake the notions that the world is being dismantled, its edges unraveling.

Sometimes your husband knows before you do. He's noted a certain posture in your sleep and a slowness in your reasoning. Your sister hears it in your legato voice: There's not melody, she says, you've gone flat. Then a glass slides from your hand. You mail your wallet.

Warning. If you're in the supermarket, abandon the shopping cart. Drive directly home. Narrate out loud: green means go. Red means stop.

Your body is a miser now, retaining fluids, keeping all to itself. Your face turns pale as milk, and half-moon circles, blue like bruises, appear under your eyes.

Next, you experience "aura," a complex neurologic mischief. The brain has a fine time of it—entertaining you or terrifying you, depending on your disposition. With the right attitude, you can traipse along, admiring the chicanery of your cortex. Consider *Alice Through the Looking Glass,* for instance, a fantasy based on Lewis Carroll's migrainous visual disturbances. Carroll perceived distortions of size: Lilliputian (diminution), Brobdingnagian (enlargement), and zoom vision.

The religious visionary Hildegarde didn't see "The Fall of the Angels" or "the Living Light." "The Aedification of the City of God?" Hardly. Yet these visions were real; so was the lightning in my eyes. The scotoma of migraine is measurable as swarms of phosphenes cross the cortical field.

During aura, you might, as I once did, get lost in a building where you've worked for a year. You wander the halls. Just where is that office of yours? It takes an hour to find. Then you close and lock the door, turn off the lights, and ring your husband, relieved to have mastered the complex trigonometrics of dialing a phone. The husband who answers is yours, though you can't quite place his first name.

You request the television be turned off with the words "Petal shower ringing."

Your vision narrows, as though you are viewing things through the wrong end of binoculars.

You don't know the year, your address, who the president is.

You look in the mirror and are shocked: your eye has moved. On closer inspection, your whole face has been segmented and rearranged. You're a living portrait conceived by a cubist painter.

Only after your brain shows off, establishing who is in charge, do you move to the next stage, with its nausea and vomiting; sensitivity to light, sound, and smell, and the legendary headache. To imagine the severity of the pain, consider the age-old remedies for it. They purge you, bleed you, lobotomize you, chop a chunk from an artery, drill a hole in your scalp. They loop a hangman's noose around your skull or anoint you with moss from a statue's head. They bind to your brow a clay crocodile stuffed with magic herbs.

And none of it helps.

Migraine resolves when your body becomes generous once more. You urinate copiously, then receive a gift of sleep. Some migraineurs are exhausted after an attack. Many, like me (also Freud, who credited his good health to "the regulatory effects of a slight migraine on Sundays"), are renewed. We appreciate. We see clearly. We get a lot done.

While writing this, I am downed. My husband and I are supposed to make a weekend foray, but we defer to my defective neurons instead. A different journey begins. Chris comes quietly into the room, offering crackers and Coca-Cola.

The weekend drones on and on. "And screen'd in shades from day's detested glare," says Pope, "She sighs forever on her pensive bed, Pain at her side, and megrim at her head."

I am not only sick, I am guilty. This is my fault, I know. Haven't the pundits—from Pliny the Elder to Aretaeus the Cappadocian, all those Romans and Greeks, the pitiless Victorians—told me it is? This "mygrame and other euyll passyons of the head" is due to my bilious humours, my hereditary taint, a hysteria of my uterus. My nervestorm is caused by masturbation, violent passions, and errors of diet. Experts of the 1930s note my retarded emotional makeup: I am perfectionistic, inflexible, and obsessive. By the late fifties, though my sins of ambition and rigidity are set in stone, I'm no longer bereft of charm. The oft-quoted Alvarez describes the small trim body, firm breasts, stylish dress, quick movements, luxuriant hair, and eager mind of the female migraineur. "These women age well," he insists.

There is comfort in the conviction that you can cure your disease by refashioning your personality. If I simply become more easygoing, I think, if I don't push so hard or stay up so late . . . but today's research dashes these hopes.

Migraine strikes the indolent as often as the driven, the sloppy along with the neat, the profligate with the parsimonious. It's an organic dysfunction, and like all biochemical disorders, it's poorly understood. Essentially, migraineurs don't have effective brain filters. Our volume controls are turned up, and we let in static. This makes the hypothalamus get kooky, alarming the reptilian brain and flustering the limbic system. Circuits break, sparks fly, and neurotransmitters run amok. The poets of medicine call it the chain reaction, the cascade, the avalanche activated when we encounter any number of everyday "triggers."

Say, for instance, that you're driving at night in a snowstorm. Your headlights illuminate swirling flakes, which seem to give birth to a million fireflies. You step on the gas and these icy stars part like a fast-forward film of the big bang theory. Bang. Big bang. This is a visual trigger that can bring on a migraine.

Or you're caught in the California Santa Anas. You face the Argentine zonkas or the Swiss foehns. These dangerous hot winds are migraine triggers all (Go to France or Canada, instead. The cool mistrals and chinooks have no effect.)

Say you forget to eat. Or you drink red wine.

And remember, someone once told me, to avoid the three c's: cheese, chocolate, and citrus. Of course, spurn the vile potato and the wicked garbanzo bean. Consume no bits of bacon, bites of hot dog, or slices of pumpkin pie.

Also thought to bring on migraine: too much sleep, too little sleep, lights, glare, altitude, stress, sex, garlic, smells, noises, humidity, travel. . . .

You may agree to give up Chianti and sauerkraut, but no vermicelli alla puttanesca. Not Argentina. Not sex. The world causes migraines, and who wants to avoid the world?

So you outwit it. The pharmaceuticals you use are beta *blockers,* calcium channel *blockers, anti*serotonins, *anti*histimines, *anti*convulsants, *anti*depressants. The self-help books are entitled *Overcoming . . . Fighting . . . Beating . . . Victory Over Migraine*—as though, in order to live, you must do battle with your own brain.

But still the hot neural storm disrupts your life, like a twister uprooting a tree— maybe not four times a week, but twice a month. In moderation, you can accept the brain's imperialism. You can stand back and watch your mind build its cathedrals.

Six or seven years old, I am sitting on the sidewalk with my cousin Sharry. The steps are cracking, and pieces of chipped cement sparkle like little gems. Then, a shift, as if a cloud has covered the sun. I look at the large, tall trees spread evenly across the lawn. I want to name them, bring to mind the sound that will tell their shape, their smell, their distinctive color. But the words, which I knew minutes ago, are no longer available. A shiver. A veil descends. I am trapped in a small, thin, mosquito-bitten body. Whose? I don't know. I've lost acquaintance with myself, but gained an opening to the unknown. I'm curious about the disposition of my soul, though I'm too young to put it that way. "Who *am* I," I say to my cousin without a question mark. I mean so much. But she laughs, expecting a foolish childhood game.

I was experiencing *jamais vu,* a sense of unfamiliarity, of a newly made world, a phenomenon, like *deja vu,* common in migraine aura. The incident so affected me that I wrote about it repeatedly as a child, until years later I found out it was simply a neurologic trick. But by then it was too late. The episode had been infused with meaning. Dutiful student of my cortex, I wondered, what am I to make of this? I learned that reality was not stable: it was subject to improvisation. I learned I could be exiled from my own life. I learned I was different from my cousin Sharry—isolated, a drifting spirit. So where did the pathology of migraine end and the development of personality begin?

Oliver Sacks, writer and doctor, calls migraine aura a veritable "encyclopedia of neurology," with its aphasias, paresthesias, paralysis, odor hallucinations, and amnesias—but it is much more. Aura delivers a whispered message of deep personal significance, more eloquent than language, more urgent than reality.

It's summer in North Carolina. Chris, Richard, and I are driving in the mountains. As we pass a town bathed in sun, sunk in a valley, I begin to feel its rhythms, its nine to five, its peculiar, humming pulse, its wooden floors grooved with a hundred years of use. It's as if its collective memory has been installed in me.

At a stop, I look at a billboard. Something is awry, undone. I can't read. I try to sound out words, concentrating like a first grader for whom each letter is a new challenge. But if I look at one part of a word, another disappears. Soon, I see the problem: there's a hole in the world and whatever I observe falls into it. My very gaze is fatal.

I touch my cheek and lips, rub my fingers together, and brush my hand down my arm. A weather front is spreading through my body, numbing one side of it. For a moment, I wonder if I've had a stroke, but dismiss this as too theatric. And though I'm not sure, I barely recall—haven't I taken similar journeys of mind before?

At a stream, Richard and Chris disappear with fly-fishing gear. I move toward the sound of water. The vegetation is lush, and though there's nowhere to sit on the bank, I see a huge boulder in the stream. I long for this rock and wade out unsteadily, conscious of a dizzying sweep of water.

I climb onto granite: solid, steady, old as the continent. It's been a long week. Chris and I have been sharing a beach house with our old friends, Rich and Carol, who are smoking again. Their children have become restless toddlers. The oldest holds her little sister's hand in a door and slams it shut; the youngest grabs shrimp off our dinner plates. It's been hot, and I haven't slept well.

But here, the air is cool, and this moment a ballet—me pirouetting on a rock, the water twirling and upstream, Richard and Chris on the water, casting, happy to be together. Suddenly it's quite clear: I've seen this exact dance before. Perhaps I've even rehearsed it. All our steps have been precisely and lovingly choreographed. It's a work of art, orderly and resolute. This is its performance.

Now I get close to the stone, feel its warmth on my cheek as I stretch across it. Soon, the pain will come, with its paralyzing but cleansing purity, and then sleep. When I awake, the sun will be in a different place in the sky. I'll be grateful for good friends and their children. My eyesight will be renewed; the edges of my life newly distinct. And though the potent elixir of knowing more than I am meant to will have disappeared, the memory of it will linger. The world will be magical and mysterious. After all, I've been its creator today: I've visited a variation of it—remade by my own mind.

Migraine

BRIAN TIERNEY

It starts at the end; the lights of cars

distorted to a burst, for a second

like asterisks, or seraph wings, extravagant & huge

as they pass me

in the exhausted sweep of fog over Mars, PA, then Punxsutawney

Parish, & New Stanton, though it's no heaven

here—the Turnpike in the rain. Cars pass & continue to

pass, & soon will arrive,

some of them, in Breezewood or Erie, where their lives have been
decided by now.

So my eyes sting *O, The Glory* & go dead. I pull over

outside Somerset; there's a rodent broke-open, a pomegranate

to the butt of a hammer, its head

useless, even to birds. It hurts to look at,

as in blood-phlegm coughed up in a bathtub. Only the body knows.

My old man, the story goes,

right before he died, he shouldered the Windstar, pulled over

to phone her, me, anyone

on his way somewhere East of

Poquessing, a faint, red fingertip print smeared on the dash

as though someone had crushed a clover mite.

Migraine

Aura and Aftermath

CLAUDIA EMERSON

First, part of the world disappears. Something
is missing from everything: the cat's eye,
ear, the left side of its face; two fingers
from my right hand; the words from the end
of a sentence. The absence is at first
more absolute than whatever darkness
I imagine the blind perceive. Perfect,
without color or motion, nothing replaces

what is gone. The senses do not contradict. My arm
goes numb, my leg. Though I have felt the cold air
of this disappearance before, each time the aura
deceives me to believe reality itself
has failed. I fear this more than what it warns
because I cannot remember I will survive it.

The other half of me will shine all night,
defined by the eclipse.
Then, in the relieved
wake of the day that follows it, I will
find my hand, count my fingers, and beginning
to see again, will recognize myself
restored to the evening of a righted room.

The Headache

Headaches

MARILYN HACKER

Wine again. The downside of any evening's
bright exchanges, scribbled with retribution:
stark awake, a tic throbs in the left temple's
site of bombardment.

Tortured syntax, thorned thoughts, vocabulary
like a forest littered with unexploded
cluster bombs, no exit except explosion
ripping the branches.

Stacks of shadowed books on the bedside table
wall a jar of Tiger Balm. You grope for its
glass netsuke hexagon. Tic stabs, dull pain
supercedes voices,

stills obsessive one-sided conversations.
Turn from mouths you never will kiss, a neck your
fingers will not trace to a golden shoulder.
Think of your elders—

If, in fact, they'd died, the interlocutors
who, alive, recede into incoherence,
you would write the elegy, feel clean grief, still
asking them questions

—though you know it's you who'd provide the answers.
Auden's *Old People's Home,* Larkin's *The Old Fools*
are what come to mind, not Yeats. In a not-so
distant past, someone

poured a glass of wine at three in the morning,
laid a foolscap pad on the kitchen table,
mind aspark from the long loquacious dinner
two hours behind her,

and you got a postcard (a Fifties jazz club)
next day across town, where she scrawled she'd found the
tail-end of a good Sancerre in the fridge and
finished the chapter.

Now she barely knows her friends when you visit.
Drill and mallet work on your forehead. Basta!
And it is *Màrgaret you mourn for* . . . Get up,
go to the bathroom.

You take the drugs. Synapses buzz and click.
You turn the bed lamp on, open a book:
vasoconstrictor and barbiturate
make words in oval light reverberate.
The sky begins to pale at five o'clock.

On a Headache

JANE AUSTEN

When stretch'd on one's bed
With a fierce-throbbing head,
Which precludes alike thought or repose,
How little one cares
For the grandest affairs
That may busy the world as it goes!

How little one feels
For the waltzes and reels
Of our Dance-loving friends at a Ball!
How slight one's concern
To conjecture or learn
What their flounces or hearts may befall.

How little one minds
If a company dines
On the best that the Season affords!
How short is one's muse
O'er the Sauces and Stews,
Or the Guests, be they Beggars or Lords.

How little the Bells,
Ring they Peels, toll they Knells,
Can attract our attention or Ears!
The Bride may be married,
The Corse may be carried
And touch nor our hopes nor our fears.

Our own bodily pains
Ev'ry faculty chains;

We can feel on no subject beside.
Tis in health and in ease
We the power must seize
For our friends and our souls to provide.

The Patient's Perspective

A Friend Like No Other

LAURIE BATITTO BISCONTI

There's a man on the couch with a
    hammer in his hand sitting next to
    me,
We are chained together,
I to him.
He to me.
There's no escape, for I do not have
    the key.
Our days and nights are spent to-
    gether as you can see,
He uses his hammer to smash my
    brain until I cannot hear and can-
    not see.
I laugh in defiance and pretend I am
    free.
But smash! Crash! Crush!
He swings his hammer again . . .
He is part of me.

There's a man on the bed with a ham-
    mer in his hand lying next to me.
I look away and wish he were gone,
But it is no use (the ice pick is on),
I wince from the blows,
Through my eyes, through my brain
    to the core of my being the ice pick
    goes.
Pain, sobs, terror flood my brain, I
    run through the house to escape
    the pain.

There's a man next to me running
    through the house with a hammer
    in his hand
He will not let me be.
Snap!
Shaking, whirling, I can feel my brain
    rattle,
The blows will not end
On goes the battle.

This is a war that will go on all night.
I have upset him somehow and I will
    give without a fight.
Down, down, crack to the floor,
The hammer explodes in my head
    with a roar.
I think to myself—"I must be no
    more."
This must be the end—the key to
    release my hammering friend.
But alas, I awake with a kick to the
    head,
I'll survive one more day,
There's pain,
I'm not dead.
I am numb now and glancing down
    at me is the man chained to me
    with the hammer striking my head,

One, two, three.
If I can only understand how he came
    to be, then perhaps I could find the
    key.
For until then, he reminds me again
    and again, that I am his prisoner,
My brain his playpen.
I can do nothing; it's up to his whim.
I retreat to the darkness, I crawl un-
    dercover but he is still with me,

A friend like no other.
The hammer swings and cracks
    through skull,
I cannot think anymore, my senses
    are dull.
There's a man chained to me with
    a hammer in his hand who has
    stolen my life,
Do you understand?

Red Migraine

MICHAEL DICKMAN

Redbreast kills
and kills itself against
the window

Sooner or later the blood in the breast will break the window into hundreds of
    pieces you can swallow whole

Keep swallowing!

Redbreast
loves you and wants you
to remember the love

So it makes you puke into the toilet blind

I was blinded by love

And drowned
in an empty bathtub
spitting up birdshit

Covered in red feathers

Sometimes redbreast likes anting with lit cigarettes safety pins paper cuts God
    that feels good

It wraps everything
in pretty pink gauze the color
of fake sunset

A pink soul

It wants to get naked and it wants it to hurt

Red teeth
Red toes
Open mouths

Who keeps pressing my head into the sidewalk

inside the bathroom

Who keeps the lights on

Who dissolves on my tongue

Who flies from my finger

Redbreast sits inside
behind your left eye
behind your right and cleans

its babies with

its beak

Scrubs its babies clean

Shakes its tail feathers to scour the floor behind your forehead and scours the
    floor red

My brain is a cutter

My initials are beats per second

Scrubbed down to zero
by the rubies
in the halo

I whispered your name into the red air

and you answered

The Headache

ROBERT HERRICK

My head doth ache,
O Sappho! take
Thy fillet,
And bind the pain,
Or bring some bane
To kill it.

But less that part
Than my poor heart
Now is sick;
One kiss from thee
Will counsel be
And physic.

Migraine

EVELYN LAU

The aura is a rumour
of thunder in the distance,
building into a storm
that rattles the shutters
and the beads of the chandelier
before punching a hole
in the load-bearing wall.

The tap of construction
through the double-glazed windows
splinters your skull.
A forty-watt bulb blazes
like an eclipse on your retina.
The faintest trace of perfume
on your wrist and throat
is a field of a thousand flowers
pumping odour.

Pain floods the house,
the chambers of your mind,
the walls swell, the ceiling hiccups
and lifts like a lid on a pot boiling over.
You are tiny in its clasp,
as in grief.
The sun rises and sets, twice.
Finally the surrender
to drugged sleep, the sweet nothing
sleep of codeine.
In the absence of feeling,
an angels' chorus.

I Describe a Migraine

IMAN MERSAL

I wanted to describe chronic migraines
as proof
that the chemical operations
in my large brain
are working in an orderly fashion.
I wanted to begin:
My hands are not enough to hold my head.
But I wrote:
a bullet from an unknown pistol tears through
a dark calm,
a great furor,
a throbbing,
the collisions of incongruous shrapnel shards.
And a pleasure too:
to excite the excruciating spots
by simply remembering them.

Migraine

JESSE PATRICK FERGUSON

Migraine:
The day's ambition pissed away.
Your bright idea an apple pricked by fly bites,
deflated beneath the sweaty palm of sunlight.

Sufferer:
Or hearing Al Purdy, mummied
in layers of cotton batting, reciting
poems in a room down the hall.

Migraine:
Also, snorting a line of thumbtacks
before a quiz on the periodic table.

Sufferer:
Periodically suspecting a wrecking ball's
begun demolishing my childhood home.
You tinker with my forehead's thermostat
until I forget the feel of my mother's hand.

Migraine:
Touching, but more like replacing the tulips'
palette with the colour of a foot
beneath a blanket in the morgue.
Listen, the mortician forgot his key in the door.

Sufferer:
And also what makes *The Price is Right*
always wrong, closes my ears to the empty
promises of daytime TV. Infomercials that blur

at their edges. The remote
impossibly far off at the foot of the couch.

Migraine:
Two extra-strength *I told you sos*
with not a glass of water in sight.
And don't forget the little flashing lights
that signal turbulence in your peripheral vision.

Sufferer:
I'd have to add: adds a twist
to the old head-in-a-vice cliché.
Headache's crazy twin kept chained
in a dark corner of the occipital lobe.

Migraine:
Agreed, and also makes a Third World
of the mind, chasing your loved ones
around unreal refugee camps.

Sufferer:
But I hate to inform you: makes me a boor
on whom all clever metaphors are lost.

Migraine:
Yes, but it's hard to lose a hairy clog
in the brain's plumbing, on a civic holiday, no less.

Sufferer:
Yes, all of these and worse—on my way
to getting fed, paid or laid, whatever,
whatever, and whatever some more.

The Voice

JOHN FULLER

I am the pulse of a new language,
The code of the invader.

I am the touch of white,
And thus I ask admittance.

I am the trace of a dim thunder,
The fear of the sentry.

I am the sound of black,
And thus I enter.

I am the dead kiss of damage,
The voice of the rebel.

I am the taste of red.
And thus I establish myself.

I am the reign of the little robbers,
The struggle of the settler.

I am the birth of pain,
And this is my time.

I am the breath of the heavy lover,
The stillness of the occupied.

I am the smell of death,
And I shall leave as I have entered.

When Nietzsche Wept

IRVIN D. YALOM

Next, a careful medical history: the patient's childhood health, his parents' and siblings' health, and an investigation of all other aspects of his life—occupational choice, social life, military service, geographic moves, dietary and recreational preferences. Breuer's final step was to allow his intuition full rein and to make all other inquiries that his data thus far suggested. Thus, the other day, in a puzzling case of respiratory distress, he had made a correct diagnosis of diaphragmatic trichinosis by inquiring into the thoroughness with which the patient cooked her smoked salt pork.

Throughout this procedure, Nietzsche remained deeply attentive: indeed, he nodded appreciatively at each of Breuer's questions. No surprise, of course, to Breuer. He had never encountered a patient who did not secretly enjoy a microscopic examination of his life. And the greater the power of magnification, the more the patient enjoyed it. The joy of being observed ran so deep that Breuer believed the real pain of old age, bereavement, outliving one's friends, was the absence of scrutiny—the horror of living an unobserved life.

Breuer *was* surprised, however, at the complexity of Nietzsche's ailments and at the thoroughness of his patient's own observations. Breuer's notes filled page after page. His hand began to weary as Nietzsche described a gruesome assemblage of symptoms: monstrous, crippling headaches; seasickness on dry land—vertigo, disequilibrium, nausea, vomiting, anorexia, disgust for food; fevers, heavy night sweats which necessitated two or three nightly changes of nightshirt and linen; crushing bouts of fatigue which at times approximated generalized muscular paralysis; gastric pain; hematemesis; intestinal cramps; severe constipation; hemorrhoids; and disabling visual problems—eye fatigue, inexorable fading of vision, frequent watering and pain in his eyes, visual blurring, and great sensitivity to light, especially in the mornings.

Breuer's questions added a few more symptoms Nietzsche had either neglected or been reluctant to mention: visual scintillations and scotomata, which often preceded a headache; intractable insomnia; severe nocturnal muscle cramps; generalized tension; and rapid, inexplicable mood shifts.

Mood shifts! The words Breuer had been waiting for! As he had described to Freud, he always sniffed for a propitious point of entry into patient's psychological state. These "mood shifts" might be just the key that would lead to Nietzsche's despair and suicide intention!

Breuer proceeded gingerly, asking him to elaborate on his mood shifts. "Have you noticed alterations in your feelings which seem related to your illness?"

Nietzsche's demeanor did not change. He seemed unconcerned that this question might lead into a more intimate realm. "There have been times when, on the day before an attack, I have felt particularly good—I have come to think of it as feeling *dangerously good.*"

"And after the attack?"

"My typical attack lasts from twelve hours to two days. After such an attack, I generally feel fatigued and leaden. Even my thoughts are sluggish for a day or two. But sometimes, especially after a longer attack of several days, it is different. I feel refreshed, cleansed. I explode with energy. I cherish these times—my mind swarms with the rarest of ideas."

Breuer persisted. Once he found the trail, he did not easily give up the chase. "Your fatigue and the leaden feeling—how long do they last?"

"Not long. Once the attack lessens and my body belongs to itself again, I assume control. Then I will myself to overcome the heaviness."

Perhaps, Breuer reflected, this might be more difficult than he first thought. He would have to be more direct. Nietzsche, it was clear, was not going to volunteer any information about despair.

"And melancholia? To what extent does it accompany or succeed your attacks?"

"I have black periods. Who has not? But they do not have *me*. They are not of my illness, but of my being. One might say I have the courage to have them."

Breuer noted Nietzsche's slight smile and his bold tone. Now, for the first time, Breuer recognized the voice of the man who had written those two audacious, enigmatic books concealed in his desk drawer. He considered, but only for a moment, a direct challenge to Nietzsche's ex-cathedra distinction between the realms of illness and being. And that statement about having the courage to have black periods, what did he *mean* by that? But patience! Best to maintain control of the consultation. There would be other openings.

Carefully, he continued. "Have you ever kept a detailed diary of your attacks—their frequency, their intensity, their duration?"

"Not this year. I've been too preoccupied with momentous events and changes in my life. But last year I had one hundred and seventeen days of absolute incapacitation and almost two hundred days in which I was partially incapacitated—with milder headaches, eye pain, stomach pain, or nausea."

Here were two promising openings—but which to follow? Should he inquire about the nature of those "momentous events and changes"—surely Nietzsche was referring to Lou Salomé—or strengthen the doctor-patient rapport by being empathic? Knowing that it was impossible to have *too* much rapport, Breuer chose the latter.

"Let's see, that leaves only forty-eight days without illness. That is a very little 'well' time, Professor Nietzsche."

"Thinking back over several years, rarely have I had times of well-being that have persisted for over two weeks. I think I can remember each one of them!"

Hearing a wistful, forlorn tone in Nietzsche's voice, Breuer decided to gamble. Here was an opening that could lead directly into his patient's despair. He put down his pen and, in his most earnest and professionally concerned voice, remarked, "Such a situation—the majority of one's days a torment, a handful of healthy days a year, one's life consumed by pain—seems a natural breeding place for despair, for pessimism about the point of living."

Nietzsche stopped. For once he did not have a ready answer. His head swayed from side to side as if he were pondering whether to permit himself to be consoled. But his words said something else.

"Undoubtedly that is true, Doctor Breuer, for some people, perhaps for most— here I must defer to your experience—but it is *not* true for me. Despair? No, perhaps once true, but not now. My illness belongs to the domain of my body, but it is not *me*. I am my illness and my body, but they are not me. Both must be overcome, if not physically, then metaphysically.

The Hangover

On His Heid-ake

WILLIAM DUNBAR

My heid did yak yester nicht,
This day to mak that I na micht.
So sair the magryme dois me menyie,

Perseing my brow as ony ganyie,
That scant I luik may on the licht.

And now, schir, laitlie eftir mes
To dyt thocht I begowthe to dres,
The sentence lay full evill till find,
Unsleipit in my heid behind,
Dullit in dulnes and distres.

Full oft at morrow I upryse
Quhen that day my curage sleipeing lyis.
For mirth, for menstrallie and play,

For din nor danceing nor deray,
It will not walkin me no wise.

My head did ache last night,
Today I can't write poetry.
So painfully the migraine does disable
  me,

Piercing my forehead like an arrow,
That I can scarcely look at the light.

And now, sire, a little after mass,
Though I tried to start writing,
The sense was difficult to find,
Deep down sleepless in my head,
Dulled in dullness and distress.

Very often at dawn I arise
When that day my spirit is still sleeping.
Neither for mirth, or minstrelsy and
  play,
Nor for noise or dancing or revelry,
It will not awaken in me at all.

Void and Compensation (Migraine)

MICHAEL MORSE

for Allen Grossman

Here's a side effect that's very front and center:
I am forgetting the words for things. It's not a matter

of mistaking the Ash for the Linden, of conjuring
the chickadees to my hand from the Arrowwood.

They are a certain kind of medicine like the image
of the beech leaves moving in a wind I cannot hear.

My head-hurt, that crush of pebbles in a tin pan,
it's still for the moment—but not my forgetting.

That's closer to home—opaque and gauzy-drunk.
There is a bowl in the dish drain; it has holes in it.

I use it to wash the greens that come out of the ground.
I use it to let water run away.

What do you call that drain inside the other drain?
Words arrive like spores from other worlds tried on and out.

And although I talk to myself like snow
in evergreens or blackbirds on wires

I know not what I'm looking through to see—
This help I need, in deed, in trust—what is it called?

I'm reading a poet who is building a boat for his death—
in love with his fading mind and what he has left of it.

PART II

What People Don't See

The Invisibility of Migraine

Introduction

The works in this part express the frustration, weariness, and progressive silence and isolation so many migraineurs share: so much of the disease is invisible, often leaving the sufferer alone with the pain of the headache and the many other invisible symptoms of the disease—the sudden mood changes (crying, irritability, loss of temper), confusion, memory problems, sudden blanks in thought or word choice, clumsiness, uncontrollable yawning, nausea, dizziness, heightened senses, and overwhelming fatigue.

Seventeenth-century poet Jane Cave Winscom suffered through endless treatments for her "headaches"; it is in her poem "The Head-Ache, or an Ode to Health" that she reminds us that migraine and its impacts can render the migraineur silent. We also realize in her poetry that she understood what every migraineur knows—its invisibility to others. Elizabeth McKim, in her insightful article "Making Poetry of Pain: The Headache Poems of Jane Cave Winscom," suggests that the poet's "primary purpose is to communicate that the devastating pain she experiences is destroying her life, and [it's] through her poems, she successfully articulates the invisibility of head pain, its silencing of the sufferer, and her anguished isolation."[1]

Families, friends, and even medical personnel will appreciate Michael Cunningham's depiction of Virginia Woolf in his book *The Hours,* which re-creates, in part for a contemporary world's perspective, Woolf's book *Mrs. Dalloway.* The interior voice of Woolf, which Cunningham communicates, not only captures the intense apprehension that Woolf feels at the prospect of her migraine returning when all she wants to do is be productive and write but also her ability to step out of her interior reverie to understand and remind herself that the struggle that she is enduring can't be seen by those around her:

First come the headaches, which are not in any way ordinary pain ("headache" has always seemed an inadequate term for them, but to call them by any other would be too melodramatic). They infiltrate her. They inhabit rather than merely afflict her, the way viruses inhabit their hosts. Strands of pain announce themselves, throw shivers of brightness into her eyes so insistently she must remind herself that others can't see them.[2]

The disease itself has no external signs, other than constricted eyes, the look of exhaustion, and the migraineur's constant pressing of muscles and trigger points that carry the pain.

Then, of course, there are the difficult side effects from the multitude of preventative, acute, and rescue medications, most of which alter the sufferer physically and emotionally in ways others can't always see or know. While friends, family, and colleagues may see the results of the medications' side effects (weight gain, mood change, unusual fatigue, confusion, difficulty focusing, memory problems), they are largely unable to recognize that these side effects are a necessary evil of living with migraine. Since so many features of migraine are invisible, all of those involved in the life of this person can learn about the diverse characteristics and bear witness. Sallie Tisdale reminds us:

> When people say they have a migraine, they usually mean a severe and peculiar kind of headache: throbbing, one-sided, accompanied by nausea and sometimes vomiting, by photophobia (oversensitivity to light) and sometimes phonophobia (oversensitivity to sound).... About 20 percent of attacks start with "auras," which range from the perception of vivid and "scintillating" lights to tingling or numbness along the skin, food cravings, trouble speaking or hearing, or depression. Some people yawn irresistably.[3]

If you are an employer, a colleague, or a physician, reading these works will help you better understand these "invisible" but often debilitating symptoms and side effects that accompany migraine. Medical professionals need to recognize and empathize with the ways in which the invisibility of this disease further complicates all aspects of a sufferer's life: it is life changing and inevitably triggers all kinds of emotional distress. The invisibility of this emotional component of the disease makes it even more vital that doctors ask the right questions to help a migraineur address these additional aspects of migraine.

A study completed by the *American Journal of Occupational Therapy* determined that:

> participants experienced major alterations in their lives as a result of chronic pain. The life changes noted by participants affect different aspects of their lives, including psychological state, occupational performance, relationships with others, and life satisfaction ... many felt emotionally overwhelmed ... experienced anxiety and fear.[4]

Margaret Vickers's *Work and Unseen Chronic Illness* speaks to how a migraineur suffers acutely in the workplace environment because her ability to mask symptoms causes her coworkers to think and say, "If you look well, you must be well."[5] Of course there is always the fear that one's work performance will suffer or will be perceived as inadequate.

Over and over again, you'll read about migraineurs who share many of the less obvious features of this disease and, too, share the exasperation and defensiveness they live with, which can only be helped by more awareness and less judgment, but the stigma remains. Edward Lowbury very accurately and succinctly captures the indifference of the general public to the predicament of the migraineur:

> Hoofbeats in the head—the nightmare's return
> With a flurry of sparks, a cloud of graveyard thoughts;
> The mind shrinks from a blank cemetery of noughts
> And crosses. People watch, but it's not their concern.[6]

Frequently, symptoms are misunderstood. While a migraineur privately experiences cognitive problems, many people often interpret such behavior either as "high" or "spacey." Joan Didion's seminal essay, which begins this anthology, poignantly captures the cognitive dimension: "I will drive through red lights, lose the house keys, spill whatever I am holding, lose the ability to focus my eyes or frame coherent sentences, and generally give the appearance of being on drugs, or drunk. The actual headache, when it comes, brings with it chills, sweating, nausea, a debility that seems to stretch the very limits of endurance. That no one dies of migraine seems, to someone deep into an attack, an ambiguous blessing."[7]

NOTES

1. Elizabeth McKim, "Making Poetry of Pain: The Headache Poems of Jane Cave Winscom," *Literature and Medicine* 24, no. 1 (2005): 93–108.
2. Michael Cunningham, *The Hours* (New York: Farrar, Straus and Giroux, 1998), 79.
3. Sallie Tisdale, "An Uncommon Pain: Living with the Mystery of Headache," *Harpers*, May 2013, 4.
4. Grace S. Fisher, Linda Emerson, Camille Firpo, Jan Ptak, Jennifer Wonn, and Gwen Bartolacci, "Chronic Pain and Occupation: An Exploration of the Lived Experience," *American Journal of Occupational Therapy* 61 (2007): 294.
5. Margaret Vickers, *Work and Unseen Chronic Illness: Silent Voices* (London: Routledge, 2001), 5.
6. Edward Lowbury, ed., *Nightride and Sunrise* (Aberystwyth: Celtion Publishing, 1978), 9.
7. Joan Didion, "In Bed," in *The White Album* (New York: Farrar, Straus, and Giroux, 1979), 170–71.

The Head-Ache, or an Ode to Health

JANE CAVE WINSCOM

AH! why from *me* art thou for ever flown?
Why deaf to every agonising groan?
Not *one* short month for ten revolving years,
But pain within my frame its sceptre rears!
In each successive month full *twelve* long days
And tedious nights my sun withdraws his rays!
Leaves me in silent anguish on my bed,
Afflicting all the members in the head;
Through every particle the torture flies,
But centres in the temples, brain, and eyes;
The efforts of the hands and feet are vain,
While bows the head with agonising pain;
While heaves the breast th' unutterable sigh,
And the big tear drops from the languid eye.
For ah! my children want a mother's care,
A husband too should due assistance share;
Myself, for action formed, would fain through life
Be found th' assiduous, valuable wife;
But now, behold, I live unfit for aught;
Inactive half my days except in thought,
And this so vague while torture clogs my hours,
I sigh, 'Oh, 'twill derange my mental powers,
Or by its dire excess dissolve my sight,
And thus entomb me in perpetual night!'

Ye sage physicians, where's your wonted skill?
In vain, the blisters, boluses and pill;
Great Neptune's swelling waves in vain I tried,
My malady its utmost power defied;
In vain, the British and Cephalic Snuff,

All patent medicines are empty stuff;
The lancet, leech, and cupping swell the train
Of useless efforts, which but give me pain;
Each art and application vain has proved,
For ah! my sad complaint is not removed.

The Hours

MICHAEL CUNNINGHAM

She looks at the clock on the table. Almost two hours have passed. She still feels powerful, though she knows that tomorrow she may look back at what she's written and find it airy, overblown. One always has a better book in one's mind than one can manage to get onto paper. She takes a sip of cold coffee, and allows herself to read what she's written so far.

It seems good enough; parts seem very good indeed. She has lavish hopes, of course—she wants this to be her best book, the one that finally matches her expectations. But can a single day in the life of an ordinary woman be made into enough for a novel? Virginia taps at her lips with her thumb, Clarissa Dalloway will die, of that she feels certain, though this early it's impossible to say how or even precisely why. She will, Virginia believes, take her own life. Yes, she will do that.

Virginia lays down her pen. She would like to write all day, to fill thirty pages instead of three, but after the first hours something within her falters, and she worries that if she pushes beyond her limits she will taint the whole enterprise. She will let it wander into a realm of incoherence from which it might never return. At the same time, she hates spending any of her cogent hours doing anything but writing. She works, always, against the fear of relapse. First come the headaches, which are not in anyway ordinary pain ("headache" has always seemed an inadequate term for them, but to call them by any other would be too melodramatic). They infiltrate her. They inhabit rather than merely afflict her, the way viruses inhabit their hosts. Strands of pain announce themselves, throw shivers of brightness into her eyes so insistently she must remind herself that others can't see them. Pain colonizes her, quickly replaces what was Virginia with more and more of itself, and its advance is so forceful, its jagged contours so distinct, that she can't help imagining it as an entity with a life of its own. She might see it while walking with Leonard in the square, a scintillating silver-white mass floating over the cobblestones, randomly spiked, fluid but whole, like a jellyfish. "What's that?" Leonard would ask. "It's my headache," she'd answer. "Please ignore it."

Pain Has an Element of Blank

EMILY DICKINSON

Pain has an element of blank;
It cannot recollect
When it began, or if there were
A day when it was not.

It has no future but itself

Its infinite realms contain
Its past, enlightened to perceive

New periods of pain.

An Uncommon Pain

Living with the Mystery of Headache

SALLIE TISDALE

"I'm very brave generally," he went on in a low voice:
"only today I happen to have a headache."
  —Tweedledum

My headache began on a Monday afternoon around three o'clock. The pain centered on my left temple and eye, constant gnawing, broken only by sudden waves of sharper pain. My doctor was on vacation, but after several days I decided I couldn't wait and took the next available appointment. By the time I made it to her office I could hardly walk across the room in a straight line.

The physician's assistant was attentive, working down the neurological checklist: reflexes, balance, gait, grip strength, and cranial-nerve function, which affects swallowing, eye movement, sensation, facial expression, and more. Everything was normal, except for the pain. Finally, with a grunt of satisfaction, she decided that I must be dehydrated. I knew that I was dehydrated because I couldn't eat because I had a headache that would not stop. By then the headache had so eroded my ability to think that I didn't even comment; I just waited in a darkened room while she wrote a prescription for Vicodin.

When my doctor returned a week later, she was also attentive, and took her time: reflexes, balance, gait, grip strength, cranial-nerve function. The Vicodin had given me no relief. I was tremulous, ill defined. The feeling was hard to describe; my words failed, trailing off.

"I'm sure it's not migraine," she told me. Migraines rarely last more than a few days. "But I'm not sure what it is." Although severe headaches are only rarely a sign of something dire, like a ruptured aneurysm or a brain tumor, she recommended an MRI to be sure.

"There is a medication that sometimes works for headaches like these," she said, and suggested I try indomethacin, an anti-inflammatory drug in the same class as ibuprofen. Usually reserved for arthritis, it's a nasty medication, known for causing stomach ulcers and gastrointestinal bleeding, cardiac arrhythmia and heart failure. I started taking twenty-five milligrams twice a day—started as soon as the pharmacist handed me the bottle—along with a daily dose of omeprazole, an acid-reducing drug, to protect my gut. The pain retreated but didn't disappear. I complained in private but mostly I kept my headache to myself, shivering my way through conversations. I had work and a class to teach and my son was getting married in a month.

Headaches are nothing special. They grant one only brief and local respite. That this one endured, that it buffeted my every step, was hard to explain. I wasn't sure anyone would believe me; after all, I hadn't really believed in such a thing, either. Another person's pain, writes Elaine Scarry, is "vaguely alarming yet unreal," and the inability to truly sympathize with another's suffering is a sign of "pains triumph." She adds, "Whatever pain achieves, it achieves in part through its unsharability."

The MRI rooms were spacious and cool. I exchanged my shirt for a cotton gown that smelled of sunshine. A young woman called my name, introduced me to a bearded man seated in front of a set of screens and led me to the machine. She deftly inserted an IV needle into my arm and slid me in. Many people feel claustrophobic in the sleek white tube of the MRI machine; I was relieved simply to lie down and be left alone for a while. The rhythmic clangs, knocks, and thuds of the magnets were not unlike the ambient music I enjoy; the clatter was soothing, and I dozed.

After a time, the frame slid out and she injected the contrast. "If there is any pathology, this will light it up," she said, and slid me back inside.

My doctor called a few days later. The MRI was clean. No tumor, no bleeding, no stroke. Over the next few weeks, I saw a dentist, a chiropractor, a massage therapist, and a nutritionist. No one had an answer. I got confused if I tried to do more than one thing at a time, even when the pain had receded. I would sometimes find myself hunched in a chair, covering my left eye with my hand, doing nothing. I began to feel like an invalid. I was not "having headaches." I had a headache, one single unrelenting headache, drowning everything else out.

Since the earliest days of medicine, the headache has been described with respect and even awe. People have long marveled at the Catholic sweep and wretched nature of its suffering, at its ability to drive victims almost mad. Headaches seem to make people see the world differently: Lewis Carroll, Vincent van Gogh, Pablo Picasso, and Georges Seurat are all said to have had them. They are a leading reason people take sick days and a common cause of visits to the emergency room. Determining the kind of headache a patient has is one of the trickier problems facing primary-care physicians. In the sometimes tautological language of medicine, headaches are both cause and effect, symptom and disorder. Descriptions are looping, self-referential. The International Headache Society created a detailed diagnostic system in 1988, but it is the subject of ongoing debate. A fair amount of the space devoted to headaches in medical and scientific journals is given over to the reorganization of categories and nomenclature. When you're in the throes of a headache, finding your place in the subsections of diagnosis is like hiking through a junkyard.

Almost all headaches are primary, meaning they aren't caused by anything else—but it is variously the muscles, blood vessels, skin, bone, mucous membranes, and nerves that hurt. That headaches can be felt in so many ways means treatment is inevitably a little experimental. Like most pains, headaches sometimes respond to placebos. They are often treated with medications prescribed "off label"—that is, in ways the FDA has not recommended for use. There are first-line drugs and second-line drugs and why-not-give-this-one-a-try drugs, and people usually use several before finding one, or a combination, that helps: antidepressants, beta-blockers, steroids, calcium-channel blockers, anticonvulsants, antihistamines, Botox, and lidocaine are all used, along with ergot (from which LSD was first synthesized) and narcotics. (And almost all these drugs can cause headaches.) But people also prescribe for themselves: butterbur, feverfew, vitamin B2, magnesium, melatonin, kudzu, vinegar, St. John's wort, coenzyme Q10, biofeedback therapy, special diets, acupuncture, and marijuana. Everything works sometimes, for someone, somewhere, and no one can easily explain why.

The majority of headaches are tension type. They often start in the morning, just as a person is waking up. The head feels squeezed as in a vise. (How many of us have had our heads put in a vise? And yet that is the image people invariably choose.) Duller pain travels down the temples and into the neck and shoulders. Despite the name, tension-type headaches are not the result of muscle tension; indeed, there is no consistent abnormality in the muscles of the head and neck during a headache, and the pain may be the result of increased sensitization in the central nervous system. When people say, "It's just a headache," they mean that it will go away in time—but how odd that a person in good health can be brought to his knees by a puzzling, harmless occurrence of unknown cause. It is a headache—but no headache is just a headache.

Headache is a peculiar insult, an intrusion into the mind; it is inherently emotional. The pain makes it hard to think and destroys equanimity, but so does the accompanying neuronal storm. Headaches trigger a response in the emotional centers of the brain; your head is making you lose your temper, making you cry. I'm not trying to claim that the pain from a headache is worse than the pain of a broken bone or the gnaw of tumor and infection—though certain types of headache cause profound pain—but there is something fundamentally different about it, a pain benign in a technical sense, malignant in an existential one. The sufferer is oddly contracted and reduced. The word is almost unbearably banal for the metaphysical jolt and psychic crisis engendered; what we call a headache is a neurological event encompassing every part of a person: body, mind, feeling, and that ephemeral construct we call *self.*

The indomethacin tamped down my constant pain, but every hour or so I had sudden tides of sharp pain that I began to call surges. They were always on the left side of my head above the eye and in the temple, with swells of tingling and electrical sensations. They made my eye squint and blink; sometimes my jaw ached, or I found myself leaning to the left in my chair. Indomethacin is singularly diagnostic for an uncommon headache I had never heard of called hemicrania continua. Indomethacin reduces intracranial pressure, but how this relates to the pain of hemicrania is unclear. Other drugs in the same class don't help; opiates don't help, and neither do the triptans, drugs that reduce the constriction of blood vessels in the brain and help treat migraine. (No other severe headache is relieved by indomethacin alone.) So, ipso facto, hemicrania is a headache that responds to indomethacin—"responds absolutely" is the classic description; an "exquisite response" is another.

I work part-time as a nurse, and that means I'm the kind of patient politely called proactive; I was in research mode as soon as I left the office. Even with my brain off center, I spent hours in the medical library reading about what my physician called "headaches like these." The description I found—of a one-sided headache that sets in suddenly, with no apparent trigger, and doesn't go away—sounded right, though only the drug would tell. "The appropriate dose will vary," I read, scribbling notes, my head cradled in my hand. One should take whatever amount of indomethacin "results in resolution of headache." With a little trepidation, my doctor agreed to let me double my dose.

Medical diagnosis is a lot less precise than people sometimes think. Illness is just description. Things we can measure are called "signs"; things the patient feels are called "symptoms"; this more or less coherent collection of details leads to a diagnosis that may be reached by trial and error. Research on the pathophysiology of headache runs to thousands of pages a year, with few answers. Are headaches generated by the peripheral or the central nervous system? How are headaches related to the immune system? "Individuals presenting with CDH," I read in an overview of the research, are considered "among the most difficult cases" a neurologist will treat.

Chronic daily headache (CDH)—a grouping of disorders rather than a diagnosis—is a term used to describe all headaches that occur at least fifteen days each month, including the specific conditions of chronic migraine, hemicrania continua, and new daily persistent headache (NDPH). People who develop chronic headaches are at risk of having them for the rest of their lives. They may, I read, lapse from medical care, seeking high doses of narcotics or such alternative remedies as electromagnetic bracelets and colon cleansing. Others may become increasingly desperate, opting for nerve blocks—injections of steroids near major nerves. (One new treatment involves implanting electrodes in the brain via the back of the neck and connecting them to a battery implanted elsewhere in the body.) Some are unable to work again, and a few kill themselves.

NDPH is a headache that develops suddenly and never goes away; this unremitting quality is the primary symptom. One of the characteristics of NDPH is that people can pinpoint when the headache started: "patients can recall exactly what they were doing and when at the time of onset." Many people with daily headaches wait weeks or even months to see a doctor. Perhaps they are afraid of what the headaches mean, or perhaps they fear that no one will be able to offer relief.

Usually the sufferer has no history of headache, but up to 30 percent of people with NDPH have a recent history of flulike illness or an upper-respiratory infection; a statistically significant number test positive for the Epstein-Barr virus. Various biochemical markers are abnormal in sufferers of chronic headaches, though knowing that you have a glutamate-receptor disturbance, decreased blood-platelet serotonin levels, increased levels of nerve growth factor and substance P, or overactivation of the contralateral posterior hypothalamus and ipsilateral rostral pons isn't much more help than being told you have a new daily persistent headache. One theory posits a temporary malfunction of the pain-control pathway. Does this mean our normal neurological environment includes pain hidden from conscious perception—that our brains have simply evolved to protect themselves from the pain of being alive?

A few weeks after the pain began, having missed work and canceled appointments and plans, I started telling more people about the headache. Immediately the advice came. Eliminate gluten. Eliminate corn. Eliminate soy, dairy, nuts. My boss told me to take a triptan. The massage therapist digging into the knot in my neck told me I needed craniofacial manipulation. A dermatologist recommended Botox. "It *might* work," she said, "and anyway, you'd get a nice wrinkle treatment for a few months."

"Your doctor is wrong," a woman said confidently. "It's a migraine. I *know*. I have migraines."

Migraine is the second most common type of headache, though headache is only one symptom of what is sometimes called a disease and other times a disorder, a condition, a syndrome. (One specialist prefers to call migraine "a genetically unique nervous-system configuration.") People with migraines are typically called "migraineurs," as though it were a profession, or a tribe. (Not every person with migraine appreciates this conflation of patient and disease, though it seems to me that many treat migraine as a central part of their identity, like a kind of ethnicity.)

When people say they have a migraine, they usually mean a severe and peculiar kind of headache: throbbing, one-sided, accompanied by nausea and sometimes vomiting, by photophobia (oversensitivity to light) and sometimes phonophohia (oversensitivity to sound). But headache is not always the main experience of migraine and may not be present at all. About 20 percent of attacks start with "auras," which range from the perception of vivid and "scintillating" lights to tingling or numbness along the skin, food cravings, trouble speaking or hearing, or depression. Some people yawn irresistibly. During a migraine attack, people can become so confused they appear intoxicated; afterward, they may experience a sense of euphoria. But there are also bilateral migraine headaches and migraine attacks without auras, nausea, or sensory or mood changes. Some migraine attacks, mostly in children, are felt primarily in the abdomen; another type causes temporary paralysis. Migraineurs may also experience Alice-in-Wonderland syndrome, in which parts of the body seem to be of abnormal size. My friend Jeanne went blind one day from a migraine; she couldn't see normally for four months.

The Migraine Disability Assessment Scale (MIDAS) determines how much time is lost to migraine from work, schooling, household chores, family time, social time, and recreation. Migraineurs have higher rates of stroke, allergies, epilepsy, and psychiatric illness than does the population at large, and also a higher incidence of depression, anxiety, substance abuse, phobias, and panic attacks; which comes first is unknown, but early childhood trauma is more common in people with migraine. People with acute migraines are protected by federal antidiscrimination law.

The aptly named "cortical spreading depression"—a slow electrical wave flowing across the brain—may be the cause of migraine's motley symptoms. The attacks may be triggered by certain types of food, nitrates, nitrites, sulfites, lack of sleep, dehydration, stress, light, altitude, menstrual cycles, menopause, and changes in the weather. Fasting can trigger a migraine attack; thus the term "first-of-Ramadan headache." Triptans are the treatment of choice for most people with migraine attacks, and for whatever reason old-school antidepressants can also work. Migraineurs may take a preventative medication every day and use another as soon as the headache starts. (This is called abortion, or rescue.) Sleep helps, but so does vomiting. I met a woman recently who told me she had become used to disabling migraine attacks accompanied by vomiting and blurry vision. One day the aura began, and she screamed, "Goddamn it, I will not have this headache!" And the headache stopped, and she never had another migraine attack. "I do believe you can argue with your body," she told me. I am not sure you can argue with every headache.

There is yet another grouping called TAC, or trigeminal autonomic cephalalgias. (Cephalalgia is Latin for "headache.") TACs are distinguished by unilateral pain following the path of the trigeminal nerve, along the face and scalp. TACs have autonomic symptoms familiar to anyone with allergies: the eyes become red or swollen; tears flow freely; the face is red and hot. Because these are one-sided headaches, the autonomic symptoms are usually one-sided as well—one droopy eye, sweating on half of the face, a single runny nostril—almost always on the side with the pain. They can be remarkably disabling: one type, which may be triggered simply by lightly touching the cheek can occur as many as 200 times a day, with each attack lasting a few seconds to several minutes. The attacks usually continue for life.

Cluster headache is included in the TAC group. Cluster describes very sharp pains on one side of the head; they come in attacks of up to eight per day, for weeks or months at a time. A cluster headache is limited in duration, but the pain is considered one of the most severe known. They have been called suicide headaches because the pain is so intense that the sufferer will sometimes bang her head against a wall or pull out her hair, and because some people do attempt suicide.

Cluster is dramatic and uncommon. Like those of migraineurs, the brains of people with cluster headaches (who sometimes call themselves clusterheads) are microscopically different from other brains. What does it mean that a third of people with cluster headaches have brown eyes? I've found sober researchers describing people with cluster headaches as having a "leonine" appearance, as being taller than average, or as having thickened skin. A correct diagnosis, some estimates suggest, can take as long as nine years. Taking triptans and breathing high-flow oxygen are the most effective treatments for cluster headaches; hyperbaric pressure also helps. But there is growing evidence that psilocybin, LSD, and related compounds can completely eliminate cluster headaches, even at subhallucinogenic doses.

And there are rarer headaches still: the thunderclap headache that can knock a person off a chair; stabbing headaches, sometimes called icepick headaches, in the eye or temple—the stabs last for just a few seconds but come in waves, many a minute in episodes lasting for days. There are headaches caused by taking too many pain-reducing medications; the brain insists on bouncing back. A nummular headache occurs in a discrete, coin-size spot. There are headaches triggered by cold or sunshine; alarm-clock headaches that wake people up from sleep like, well, clockwork; preorgasmic headaches and orgasmic headaches and exertional headaches that make people ill when they exercise, and headaches you feel only when you cough.

None of these are my headache.

The pain of hemicrania continua centers around the eye and forehead. (A number of people with HC experience "foreign body" syndrome, the sense that there is something in the eye.) HC may seem to wax and wane, but it never disappears; in fact, it is layered: the moderate, relentless foundation, a kind of water torture of headache, overlaid with bursts of sharp, even blinding, pain. Many people with hemicrania (and "many" is the wrong word; it is rarely diagnosed, though some researchers think it is less rare than once believed) also have "migrainous" symptoms, like my occasional nausea and sensitivity to light.

How quickly I was willing to take on the risks of indomethacin! I felt dizzy, clumsy, weak, but whether this was the medication or the headache is hard to say. The continual pain faded into the background, turning into a kind of internal pressure, as though the headache were pushing on the inside of my head, trying to get out. The surges diminished in frequency, and then in the intensity, but didn't cease. Beneath the business of preparing for my son's wedding, a monotone of dull pain; on top of the happiness and cheer, the faint perfume of indomethacin. After a few weeks, I found myself sinking to the bottom of Maslow's hierarchy of needs: in danger. One night my heart began to skitter and twitch; I lay in bed and hoped they wouldn't take my medicine away.

I didn't tell my doctor about my heart, but still she refused to increase my dose, instead referring me to Dr. N., a neurologist with a weeks-long waiting list. Together they decided to start me right away on a low dose of gabapentin, an anticonvulsant. I was making the rounds that mark a long illness: telephone calls and paperwork, waiting on hold listening to pop songs and sitting in waiting rooms and waiting to make a new appointment with a front-office clerk who never makes eye contact and asks for my "social" and then interrupts me to take a phone call, and I just wanted to be able to do *something*. I was acutely aware of being the patient, of having less power than the people to whom I was explaining myself. They were well and busy and I was only a small part of their day.

Dr. N.'s office is one in a long row of anonymous medical offices beside a small hospital in a town next to Portland, Oregon. He is Indian, a small and tidy man with a light accent. When I met him, about two months after my headache began, he was attentive, walking me through the exam: reflexes, balance, gait, grip strength, and cranial-nerve function. I had been on the gabapentin a month by then; my headache was muffled, but still unrelenting.

It's not a migraine, he said dismissively. Nor is it cluster. And because I had not had an absolute—not an *exquisite*—response to indomethacin, he doubted that I had hemicrania continua. He pulled me into a dark room to show me the MRI on a computer, flipping rapidly through my brain; the lovely scalloped layers widened and thinned as we traveled through the slides. I would not have been surprised if the MRI had shown a tumor, or if my brain were lanced by the plaques of dementia. But mine was spotless, a smooth, dark-gray brain, a good-looking brain.

"See, it's clear," he said, as though we were discussing a spring sky. No clouds today. But then he pointed to a tiny spot, a small white curl of bone. "This could be it," he said. "I think this is contact point." I suspected that it wouldn't be easy to get a smile out of this guy, but he smiled then. A solution. Seven years before, I'd had surgery on my sinuses, and I might now have a little bony overgrowth as a result. A contact-point headache is secondary, caused by a pinched nerve; pain is referred along the trigeminal nerve, and usually alleviated by surgery.

We talked about my odd jitteriness, how my body felt fragile and shaky, like a poorly built scaffold beginning to lean. Was this the headache or the drugs? It was hard to tell—but he suggested that I increase my gabapentin dose quickly, that I really load up, and get off the indomethacin. This would be good for my heart. Gabapentin is a safer drug, but its side effects are varied: weakness, joint aches, depersonalization, somnolence, poor coordination, "strange feelings."

Almost immediately, my heart settled down. But that week of weaning myself off the indomethacin gave me a headache that seemed to fill the world. When

I woke each morning, I couldn't think clearly. *What time is it?* I would wonder. *What's going on?* Eventually I would rise, going straight for the morning dose, then dip my head under the faucet before climbing into the shower, pulling on clothes, and careering into the kitchen to line my stomach for the pills. Within an hour of each dose, I'd feel better. I've never needed medication in this acutely timed way before; it seemed the first sign of a fatal erosion. I resented the needing of it.

I had a CT scan and returned to Dr. F., who'd done my sinus surgery: a short, bald man with a head shaped like a ball. He perched casually on the exam table and told me that there was nothing to be seen on the CT—no bone spur, no contact point. The interventionist with tools for cutting bone didn't want to intervene, and though invasive studies and surgery are generally way down on my list of things to do, I was disappointed to tears.

So I waited three weeks for the next appointment and went back to Dr. N., who was not smiling.

"I've reached my limit on headaches," he told me. "I'm a general neurologist. If you had Parkinson's disease? Multiple sclerosis, epilepsy—that's what I do."

Having reached the mountaintop of his exam table again, I was not willing to relinquish it so quickly. "Do you think it's possible this really is a persistent headache?" I asked. NDPH: the headache that never goes away, never gets diagnosed beyond its own description, with few treatments.

He nodded. "Yes, perhaps." Precise syllables, a cock of the head.

"What about going on an elimination diet?" I asked.

He shrugged a very small, tidy shrug. "It can't hurt," he said.

In order to see a headache specialist, I had to get authorization from my insurance provider to go out of network. I have good insurance, but I was into this for thousands of dollars by then. As the bills began to arrive, I could see why people delayed treatment, or gave up. More time on the phone, more voicemails, explaining myself to the point of crying, head in hand, letters, more calls, more waiting. How do people who don't know how to work the system navigate it? How do people with *headaches* navigate it?

I had reached a point of feeling almost infinitely strange. I still had a headache all the time, though it was masked; I was depersonalized. Something almost like an aura ebbed and flowed away—the feeling of a crucial piece broken wild and loose, the cotter pin of control. After a particularly bad day, when my skin felt like fuzzy wool and I was afraid to drive, and I couldn't get an appointment with anyone, I cut back on my medication; I had plenty now, and I had reached the point of prescribing for myself. Soon my thinking cleared up, but the surges renewed—pain, and a frisson of electricity around the eye, into the cheek, a vague tingle. I found myself getting used to it.

Dr. P.'s headache clinic was just off a busy freeway exit at the junction of two overgrown suburbs of Portland, a cheap second-story office with a few small rooms and cardboard boxes piled in one corner next to a few chairs near the secretary's desk. No standing on ceremony for Dr. P., a woman shaped like an apple, with a halo of strawberry hair; she just stuck her head out of one of the rooms and called me in.

First, we talked: the entire history of the headache, my family medical history, the medications I'd taken, how I felt right then. When I tried to explain that I sometimes felt like I had a headache without actually having pain, she knew what I meant. She heard this a lot—that something feels wrong in the head in an uncertain way. All she does is headaches; the only patients she sees are patients like me, struggling to explain the way it feels inside our heads, stumbling over words because each thought is work. It was only after we had talked for forty-five minutes that she examined my reflexes, balance, gait, grip strength, cranial-nerve function.

Finally, she pressed on my shoulders for a moment and stepped back. "I'm quite sure this is hemicrania. The indomethacin didn't work perfectly because you couldn't take a high enough dose." She had seen it before. We discussed alternative drugs, one of which, topiramate, is known to cause memory and speech problems. She suggested lamotrigine, another anticonvulsant, instead, noting that I would have to increase the dose very slowly. Lamotrigine has interesting side effects—behavioral changes, nausea, double vision, and the rare Stevens-Johnson syndrome, a widespread inflammatory reaction in which large sections of skin blister and slough off. Lamotrigine can also cause headaches.

I winced at her description.

"How long do I need to take it?"

"I hope I can talk you into a year," she answered. "Sometimes hemicrania just burns itself out. Sometimes it doesn't."

The quiet paring of disease, the fraying at the edges of liver and heart, the vision slowly blurring, the cough that sticks around. Sometimes we can only rely on a kind of maladaptation. We get used to it.

All along, I have written about *my* headache, as though it were a possession, something I could grasp. This headache has been my close companion for a while now; we are intimate. I'm not a migraineur; I'm not a clusterhead. Perhaps hemicrania is not that uncommon, but I've never met anyone else who has it. That my doctor even knew enough to suspect it is to her credit; most doctors and nurses I know have never heard of it. Most have never heard of chronic daily headache, and several have asked me, "So when someone tells me they've had a headache for years, maybe I should believe them?" Yes, I say. Believe them.

I'm on a drug that is not benign; I've gained some weight, and my blood pressure has gone up a bit. I am still occasionally dizzy, and, for the first time in my life, I'm sensitive to the sun. Only months after I began taking lamotrigine did I suddenly remember that it is sometimes used for mood disorders; now and then I wonder how much of my sense of wellbeing is just the chemical. But it helps. Reading my journal from the spring, I find it hard to accept my fragile handwriting, the daily recording of what felt like slow destruction. I don't have a headache most of the time now, and not having a headache is like being twenty years younger. I have energy and good cheer and I can hike and travel. I can write again, at last. Then the surge comes. I stop, hold my hand against my temple, cupping my eye. I stand still for a moment, feeling the pain scrape across the bone above my eye and fade. And then I forget again.

Migraine

The Eternal Return

JACK SHOLL

Characters:
Friedrich Nietzsche   Philosopher
Lou Salome   Franz Nietzsche's former paramour
Overbeck   Professor of Liturgical Studies

Music: Mussorgsky's "Night on Bald Mountain"
The second-story apartment of a middle-aged Friedrich Wilhelm Nietzsche in Turin, Italy. On the right of the stage is a bed. To the left, by a door, is a wooden table and wooden chair. On the desk is a pile of papers next to an inkpot and pen. To the rear center of the stage is a wooden bureau on which sits a ceramic water pitcher and water basin, and two dozen differently colored bottles and boxes of different shapes and sizes. The walls and floor are bare. A window in the far corner rear emits light into the room. A clock tower in the plaza is visible through the window. Next to the window is a black telephone on a small table. The year is 1888.
Nietzsche, with a giant walrus mustache and swept-back hair, lies on the bed, in striped pajamas, his head propped on a pillow, his hand clutching his head.
(The telephone rings. The answering machine clicks on.) "You have reached the residence of Friedrich Wilhelm Nietzsche. No one is at home. No one will be home. Please do not call back."

NIETZSCHE: *(Writhes on the bed and moans in great pain):* Aaaaahhhhhh! Will this never cease! *(He sits up in bed and clasps his head between his hands. He gets off the bed and walks slowly to the bureau, where he mops his brow with a wet towel from the water basin. He pours a glass of liquid from one of the bottles into a glass on the bureau and drinks it down. He goes to the desk. He holds his head between his hands in agony. He writes. The room grows dark. He lights a candle on the desk. He continues to write. He returns to the bed.)*
(A knock on the door.)
NIETZSCHE: Come in. The door is unlocked.

(Lou Salome enters.).

(Nietzsche lies prostrate on the bed. Lou advances to the bed. She feels his brow.)

LOU: You have a very high fever.

NIETZSCHE: I am unable to get up.

(Lou goes to the wash basin and gets the wet towel. She returns to the bed and mops Nietzsche's brow.)

LOU: I came as soon as I got your letter.

NIETZSCHE: I am dying.

LOU: Oh, you always say that! You're not dying. I know your migraine headaches are intolerable, but you always manage to live through them.

NIETZSCHE: No. This time I know it. My horrible wracked body I know so well, my life-long tormented, painful body tells me so. I have lived with it too long to know it's not lying. And if I'm not dying, I might as well, the way I am.

LOU: Have you taken your medicines?

NIETZSCHE: Yes. They no longer help. I am taking two grams of morphine a day. Plus my other tonics, pills and elixirs. Nothing helps this endurable pain and anguish.

LOU: Should I go for the doctor?

NIETZSCHE: No. The doctor can no longer help. I called you here because before I die I must pass on my secret to someone, the secret I have worked my entire life to discover. Otherwise, it will die with me. Sit by me and listen.

(Lou sits down on the edge of the bed next to Nietzsche, who sits up next to her. He takes her hand.)

NIETZSCHE: (Quiet, matter-of-fact, but in deep horror, trembling.) We live in an indifferent universe. There's nothing. There's no God. There are no gods. It's all chance and chaos. It's all meaningless.

LOU: There must be some purpose?

NIETZSCHE: No, no, there's not. Everything, and I mean everything in the world, in the universe is energy. Organic life originates in purely random combinations. It's a giant game of dice. Everything in natural existence is an enormous interplay of dynamic and differential forces, an ever-changing aggregation and re-aggregation of forces of energy. All is energy and energy in flux. Absolutely everything is a combination of random events.

LOU: Everything? Even you and me?

NIETZSCHE: Yes. Even you and me. Everything from the tiniest to the largest. From the smallest grain of sand, and the molecules that make it up, to the largest star.

LOU: Randomness and chaos. A meaningless universe. No God. No after life. Never to smell the flowers again. Or hear the laugh of a lover's voice. How depressing.

NIETZSCHE: Not to worry, though. I've got it all figured out.

LOU: How so?

NIETZSCHE: Time is on our side. Everything comes back again. There is an Eternal Return.

LOU: What do you mean?

NIETZSCHE: Infinity. That's our wild card. We've got a finite amount of energy. Some of it is weak and some stronger. These energy forces constantly differentiate themselves into greater or lesser particular groupings of force. In an infinite amount of time, the constituent forces will recur, or return, constantly in subsequent aggregations. The sum of these natural forces is the Eternal Return. Thus, everything returns again, and again, and again. Hence, the Eternal Return is an infinite repetition of the same. Got it?

LOU: Yeah, I got it. But I fail to see where it makes any difference. If everything comes back again and again, what difference does it make? Nothing really changes. I will forever have my loss of faith. I'll still have that ugly mole on my back. And my dishpan hands.

NIETZSCHE: I have thought of this. The play of chance, with its millions of combinations of so many series, forms a chain, without beginning or end. It's really a circle. So, the good news is we can rewill ourselves at one of the repetitions.

LOU: Well, I must admit I always thought if it could be done over again, I'd like just a little more tilt to my nose.

NIETZSCHE: Communication between *inorganic* matter is simple and direct. It's all chemical codes and electrical charges—keys-in-locks, hands-in-gloves kind of stuff. *Organic* matter is another story. When *inorganic* happens to change to *organic*, watch out: a life force is developed. This life force finds it necessary to perpetuate, to create and succeed itself as a life force. The strong energy always tries to overcome the weak. The strong energy must believe in its own necessity once it becomes organic. It—energy in the sense of physics—must strive by will to the spiritual. Before, and after the organs are created. Then on to the level of the human psyche. This life force exerts a will to power. It is a human goal that occurs amid the natural forces.

LOU: What's so different about the inorganic and organic forces? What's the big difference?

NIETZSCHE: Basically, there should be no errors in communication between inorganic forces. Once we get organic communications, there is error. When there is error, there is necessity. The necessity for the strong to prevail over the weak. Errors occur when humans start to meddle. Chance is always a part of the moment of which that moment is composed. As soon as the individual exists, and understands this, the human cannot fail to rewill all the before-and-after series of its own existence.

LOU: Oh, Fred! How shall we live our lives?

NIETZSCHE: The *Ubermensch*, the overman, is the model. Above the fray, not tied to the past, forgetting about the past, strong, courageous, adventuresome, humorous. No wimps, that's for sure. If the *Ubermensch* forms himself at a juncture of the Eternal Return, from that point on it will be the *Ubermensch* who then will endlessly return forever in all future Eternal Returns *ad infinitum*. I haven't got it all figured out yet. What I can say with assurance, though, is that we must strive for the best life, because it will return over and over again. You don't want a bad one returning, now do you? We must strive to be *Ubermensch*es.

LOU: No, of course not. But listen here, Fred, if I understand you correctly, the universe is like the proverbial twelve monkeys typing endlessly on a typewriter who will eventually produce all the works of Shakespeare?

NIETZSCHE: Well, yes. I would have picked someone else, like Herodotus or Homer. But, well, yes.

LOU: Hmmm? What if those monkeys were to use one of those newfangled typewriters? It would be faster than handwriting, and dipping quill in ink and so forth. I'm speaking by analogy, of course, but if the *Ubermensch* comes along, then he or she could produce a faster process and it would diminish or shrink the times between the returns. Don't you think?

NIETZSCHE: Ah, you are Papa Nietzsche's girl, after all. You have an interesting point there. Anything that would speed up the process would speed up the iterations of the Eternal Returns, and, thus, the arrival of the *Ubermensch* to beat all *Ubermensch*es.

LOU: But, you know, Fred, even after what you've said about coming back again, and even in a more prefect state, fundamentally the universe is still meaningless, full of chaos and disorder.

NIETZSCHE: Yes, that's correct.

LOU: (Despondent.) How horrible.

(Nietzsche puts his arms around her shoulders.)

NIETZSCHE: Now, now. Don't despair. It'll be all right. It'll be OK.

LOU: (Head bowed.) Is there an answer? To a meaningless universe. (Nietzsche gets up and slowly walks across the room.)

NIETZSCHE: Yes, there's an answer.

(Nietzsche stops at the bureau. He pours draughts from several bottles into a glass and drinks it down.)

NIETZSCHE: Yes, my little wienerschniztel, there's an answer: To forget, and The Will To Power! The natural will of the strong force to prevail over the weak. *(Nietzsche does a soft-shoe dance. He takes another slug from the glass. He twirls back to the bed and sits down beside her. He takes her disconsolate face in his hands.)* NIETZSCHE: I didn't mean to distress you. It'll be OK. Relax, you'll feel better. *(eases her back onto the bed and lift her legs onto the bed.)* Everything'll be OK. *(Rests her head against the pillow and pulls the cover over her. And crawls in beside her.)* Here, here, let Papa Nietzsche tell you about the Will to Power and how the superman brings the vast, infinite flux of energy of nature to meaning. My little strudel.

(Lou bolts upright, jumps out of bed and straightens her skirt and hair.)

LOU: Hold it right here, Fred. After all, I'm a married woman!

NIETZSCHE: My little honey pot!

LOU: Keep your dirty thoughts to yourself!

NIETZSCHE: *(Grasps his head.)* Mein Lieben!

LOU: Why do you have to pick *me* to tell your secrets of the universe? Why can't you tell the world? At least some others?

NIETZSCHE: I can't, yet. To be honest, I am not yet completely, 100 percent certain. I absolutely know it; but it must be indisputably provable. Otherwise, I speak only to myself.

LOU: How will you prove it?

NIETZSCHE: I will prove it scientifically. With physics experiments.

LOU: How?

NIETZSCHE: I plan to devote ten years of exclusive study to the natural sciences at the University of Paris or Vienna. After ten years of absolute silence, I will, if I am successful, step among people again to teach the doctrine of eternal recurrence. If I am mad, science will prove me so. And then I will know that I am nothing but a poor, suffering madman. And nothing more. You have seen my suffering. You've been part of it.

LOU: Now, wait one minute! You're not going to lay this whole concept of Eternal Return on me, are you?

NIETZSCHE: You know how I suffered.

LOU: We've been through this a thousand times. Paul and I . . .

NIETZSCHE: Don't start me on that little milksop.

LOU: Oh, no matter. In case you haven't heard, I married, again.

NIETZSCHE: *(Holds his head in despair.)* Ohhhh, you would have been the center of my life!

LOU: I couldn't marry you, Friedrich. To tell you the truth, you make me nervous. In fact, very nervous. It wouldn't have worked out. Your only interest is the over-man. You think it's OK for others to have children. But not you. You yourself said that *Zarathustra* was your child.

NIETZSCHE: But that was without *you*.

LOU: Friedrich, give it a break! Don't you think I don't read everything you write?

NIETZSCHE: The only future is the child.

LOU: The future, yeah, yeah, yeah. But you've got to have a baby, Fred, spelled B-A-B-Y—kitchee, kitchee, koo!—a real, living, squealing, messy little baby to project the future. Not a book, not an abstraction, not a teaching. Do I have to quote you from memory: "I have never met a woman by whom I wanted children, unless it be you, oh Eternity." And just who wrote that, Mr. Wise Guy? To tell you the truth, Fred, if there's a child around here, it's you.

NIETZSCHE: Huh?

LOU: I mean, just look at the way you live. You're like a hobo. Traveling from one place to the next. Living in sparse rooms like an ascetic. You have no job. You're unemployed. Maybe you haven't heard, but a child, a real child, a son or a daughter, has real needs. And you need money to raise a child and a family.

NIETZSCHE: I get my royalties on my books.

LOU: Oh? And just how many copies of your latest blockbuster, *Beyond Good and Evil,* sold?

NIETZSCHE: (*Ponders for a moment.*) Three.

LOU: And who bought them?

NIETZSCHE: Me. Well, after all, 1 had to have presentation copies for Bauer, Burckhardt, and Keller.

LOU: I rest my case. Fred, have you ever thought about getting a job?

NIETZSCHE: I teach.

LOU: I mean a real job. The market for people interested in philology is rather limited, the last 1 heard.

NIETZSCHE: I teach the *Ubermensch.*

LOU: Ah, if we could only bottle it!

NIETZSCHE: Acchhh. (*Explodes.*) It was wrong of me to ask you to come. I thought if anyone could understand me, it would be you. You are like all the other addlepated cabbage heads. How much truth can a spirit *bear,* how much truth can a spirit *dare?*

I should have known better than to get involved with a smart, clever woman. Woman, know thy place! Thou art a bearer of children. And, if you're not, keep your opinions to yourself.

(*A knock on the door.*)

LOU: Let me see who it is.

NIETZSCHE: Tell them to go away. Remember my secret. Tell no one. You swear? If the rabble were to get wind of it . . .

LOU: I know, I know. I swear. (*She crosses the room and opens the door.* Franz Overbeck *enters.*)

LOU: (*Surprised.*) Why, it's you, Professor Overbeck!

NIETZSCHE: Come in, Overbeck.

OVERBECK: I understood you were very ill. I got a little worried. (*Aside to Lou.*) He signed his last letter to me "The Crucified." (*To Nietzsche.*) I came to see if there's anything I can do?

NIETZSCHE: (*Nietzsche staggers out of bed, and, in great pain, goes to Overbeck and embraces him.*) Overbeck, my old friend! (*Nietzsche bursts out crying in great sobs.*) Booohhh, hoooo, hoooo. (*Nietzsche, sobbing, lumbers back to bed, lies down, and moans.*) Ohhh. Ohhhh. Ohhh. (*Nietzsche falls asleep, snoring loudly.*)

LOU: He's mad.

OVERBECK: Of course he's mad. He's always been mad. He's thought more deeply about the human condition than anyone else, ever.

LOU: No. I mean really mad. Crazy. (*Lou circles her forefinger around her temple and whistles.*) Insane. He's gone bonkers. He's not playing with a full deck. He's finally gone over the deep edge to pure insanity.

OVERBECK: What's he been saying?

LOU: Oh, you know, the usual. Overman stuff.

OVERBECK: Ah, yes, the *Ubermensch.*

LOU: *Ubermensch, schmubermensch,* overman, superman. I tell you he's as mad as a hatter! I don't know what will happen to him.

OVERBECK: Did he say anything else?

LOU: Well, yes. But I promised I wouldn't tell.

OVERBECK: I think under the circumstances you can tell me. It may have something to do with his condition. It may enable me to help.

LOU: But I promised.

OVERBECK: Well, then, give me a hint. If I guess it, you really won't have told me. Right?

LOU: Hmmm.

OVERBECK: Oh, come on, now.

LOU: Well, OK. Let's say you left the room, went out the door and came back again. What would you have done?

OVERBECK: I would have come back.

LOU: No, no. You're warm. But not hot. Let me say it, again. You go out of the room and come back. What do you do?

OVERBECK: I re-enter the room.

LOU: (*Jumps up and down excitedly.*) No, no, no. You're burning hot. But still not there. (*Slowly.*) You go out, and you come back.

OVERBECK: I return. Oh, I get it! Of course, the Eternal Return! I return and return over and over again infinitely.

LOU: You know it?

OVERBECK: Oh yes. He shared that esoteric doctrine with me when visited him a while ago at the Croix Blanche Hotel in Basel.

LOU: (*To Neitzsche*): Why you two-timing, two-faced, lying no good for nothing! I thought I was the only one you told! I'll eternally return you!

NIETZSCHE: (*Grasping his head.*) Ohhhh! Ohhh! My head. My head. Never a moment of peace. I can hardly think!

OVERBECK: (*To Lou.*) My train leaves in several hours. Could you stay with him?

For a while? Care for him? Until he gets better?

LOU: Look, I only had a fling with him. I couldn't live with him. No one could live with him.

OVERBECK: Yes, I suppose. You've gotten back with Paul?

LOU: I've remarried, someone else. And besides, Friedrich sees woman only as a vessel for man. He doesn't take women seriously. I mean, you don't hear him carrying on about uberfraueleins, or overwomen, or superwomen, do you? *(Nietzsche leaps from the bed.)*

NIETZSCHE: Superwomen, my ass, monkey brains! There can be no superwomen. It's not in women's nature. You speak of the emancipated woman. Woman is meant to bear children. That's their only role. It's built into them physiologically. That's why they're at a disadvantage to man. They're at a medical disadvantage. The emancipated women lack the stuff for children.

(Overbeck walks to the window and stares out, his back to Nietzsche and Lou.)

In the eternal war between the sexes, nature puts woman in a superior position by far. Women don't need grammar school education. They don't need trousers or the political rights of voting cattle.

Emancipation is the instinctive hatred of the woman who has turned out ill. She's incapable of bearing a child, in opposite to the woman who has turned out well. When a woman elevates herself as a woman-in-herself, or as a higher woman, or as an idealist-woman, she lowers the general rank of woman. The more a woman is a woman, the more she defends herself against rights.

At bottom, the emancipated women are the anarchists in the world of the eternal-womanly. Emancipated women are the underprivileged whose deepest instinct is revenge against humanity.

LOU: You rule out sex and sexual pleasure?

NIETZSCHE: No, chastity is anti-nature. Contempt for the sexual life, every befouling of it though the concept impure, is *the* crime against life—is the intrinsic sin against the holy spirit of life.

LOU: *(To Overbeck.)* What do you think, Professor Overbeck? After all, you're a preacher. What do you counsel the young women of today? Free love or the eternal chains of motherhood?

OVERBECK: *(Overbeck turns from the window.)* Maybe we're just in one of those in-between periods between millennia that Friedrich always talks about. Right, Friedrich? You know, between generations, between the old and the new.

NIETZSCHE: The rabble. . . .

LOU: *(Cuts him off.)* I have news for the two of you. If you haven't noticed, women are over the hump. If anything, I'd call Mr. Friedrich Nietzsche and his *Ubermensch* the Super Kvetch. The man with the luxury to criticize everyone and anything anytime.

(Nietzsche pours a large draught from a bottle on the bureau into a glass. He downs it in one large gulp.)

OVERBECK: Let's not get into politics, my dear. After all, we're here to help Friedrich.

NIETZSCHE: *(Paces the floor animatedly, with great agitation.)* The rabble spend their lives like swine feeding at the trough of lust. Should we not create—should we not become—before we reproduce?

Our responsibility to life is to create the *higher,* not to reproduce the *lower.* Nothing must interfere with the development of the hero inside of us. And if lust stands in the way, then, it, too, must be overcome.

How does one cure—redeem—a woman? I'll tell you, cabbage head! One makes a child for her. That's how! The woman has need of children, the man is always only the means.

(Nietzsche staggers and collapses onto the bed, and drops off to sleep, snoring loudly.)

LOU: *(To Overbeck.)* I had a dream on my overnight stop here.

NIETZSCHE : *(Moans deliriously from the bed; thrashes.)* We all dream. It's the chaos pushing against the consciousness of the mind.

LOU: The dream was of a blonde, buxom, Mittel-European woman. She said she "Vants to be alone." I took it as a portent. Great artists and thinkers, like Friedrich, need peace and quiet if their great works are to flourish.

OVERBECK: We all want to be alone, sometimes. It's healthy. It's rejuvenating. It helps separate the wheat from the chaff. No human can withstand it permanently. Only the truly mad in their own universe. The autistic, for example.

LOU: He can, apparently.

OVERBECK: No, that's not what the woman in your dream meant. What she meant is to escape from celebrity. The women in your dream was no doubt an operatic diva or a theatrical actress. Friedrich's books are not, after all, exactly best sellers.

LOU: That's for sure. Only he, you, Wagner and Strindberg can understand what he's saying.

OVERBECK: No, there's something more going on here with him. Yes, Friedrich is a loner. But he sees and knows the value of others. He knows that's where the individual derives his meaning—in other individuals. His is not an unpeopled universe. Oh, maybe in his world the common rabble aren't worth associating with, but then an *ubermensch* or two, well, that's a different matter.

LOU: He said he wants to do a scientific experiment.

OVERBECK: Heh?

LOU: To prove he's right.

OVERBECK: On the Eternal Return? How's that possible? It would take lifetimes.

LOU: I told you he's nuts. He said he's prepared to spend years on it. And, get this, he doesn't even believe in science.

OVERBECK: I could have sworn he told me he sees science and technology as the new religion, replacing the old.

LOU: No, you misunderstood him. Goodness knows that's easy enough to do. He sees science and technology replacing religion, just as he sees nationalism replacing religion. He didn't say it was a good thing, or that he believed in it. He just said it was a replacement the rabble could take succor in. Just like logic, which he doesn't like, either. Oh, that's not fair. It's not logic *per se* he doesn't like. He doesn't like it as an object or process of consolation—as a mental balm or escape from the real nature of things. At bottom, science in his mind seeks to establish the way the human being in general and not the individual feels in relation to all things and to him or her self. Religion used to create and perpetuate the norms of society. Now science does it. Science creates a phantom over reality. It's an interpretive force that proves or disproves itself. It's borne out of a need to calculate. It's embedded in the mind. It's the mind endlessly chattering away—to itself or to anyone else who'll listen. It's not the physical universe *per se* at work. Remember, Professor Overbeck, we were talking about the monkeys?

OVERBECK: Yes.

LOU: Well, look at it this way. The calculation, whether done by monkey fingers, by hand or by super-*mensch* computer is the same. It's the same calculation. Fast or slow. Get it! The same calculation. Does physics follow the mathematics or does mathematics follow the physics?

OVERBECK: Aren't we playing a game of which came first. The chicken or the egg?

LOU: No. We're dealing with the biggest, smartest, and most probably overwrought brain of the 19th Century. Someone who's seen further back, and further ahead, than any human. The only comparison may be a couple of ancient Greeks and maybe, I say, maybe, Karl Marx. That's all. No other competition. Fred seriously believes science should be liberated from its social foundations. He's for the individual, at best a small group of completely independent *Ubermensche*s who will be responsible for all knowledge and scientific experimentation who'll put it to use of societies. It must be returned to the individual.

OVERBECK: Dear me! Should I throw away my new daguerreotype camera?

LOU: No, of course not. I wouldn't do that just yet. By the way, I positively adored that photo you sent us last year of you and Frau Overbeck tripping through the edelweiss in the Endigane.

OVERBECK: Why, thank you!

LOU: Don't mention it. Also, by the way, Fred thinks that the man who can fly will inherit the earth and be the most powerful person on the planet. But don't count on it. I wouldn't plan just yet on booking your next vacation to Baden-Baden by air.

OVERBECK: No problem. We'll take the train as usual. As it's oft been said, if man were intended to fly, he'd have wings.

LOU: *(Looks about suddenly.)* Oh, how impolite! What a poor host our dear Friedrich is. Would you care for something to drink, Professor Overbeck? Perhaps a schnapps?

OVERBECK: Now that sounds like a good idea. This is really starting to give me a headache. Is there any in the house?

LOU: Yes.

(She goes to the bureau top and produces a bottle of schnapps and two glasses.)

LOU: On the rocks?

OVERBECK: No, straight up.

LOU: Just as well. There's no ice anyway in this hermit's cave.

OVERBECK: Hmmm. I thought Friedrich always calleth the iceman.

LOU: He did. He drank to stop the pain of his migraines. But he gave up drinking. He said alcohol dulls his senses. You know, there's something else going on here with Friedrich. Behind that ridiculous, ponderous moustache, I just know Fred is trying to hide behind philosophy to conceal his own madness. I'm not saying Fred's mind isn't crackerjack. He's brilliant. I mean, after all, you don't think I would have gone out with just anyone? But he's put a philosophical mask over a psychological problem. He escapes to philosophy to escape from his own personal suffering of life. When you come down to it, the problem isn't philosophical after all, it's psychological. The will to be other than you are in order to become what you are. To overcommand and lose identity. The necessity for the individual to live in a series of individualities.

Fred wants to disappear. I mean, what are we talking about here with this Eternal Return? The repetition of every event, every action, every historical period, every geological epoch, every animal, every plant, and every species of every genus of animal and plant, every planet, constellation, the entire cosmos, the universe itself, every insect, every wooly mammoth, every zebra fish, duckbilled platypus, every dodo bird, emu and egret, marsupial and Komodo Dragon, every stone, every electron, proton and photon, every person, every part of a person at any time—a constant permutation or a constant permutation of things in an infinity of natural forces that give us new things in the same sequence or not. What a colossal fantasy! Is it actually possible?

OVERBECK: The accounts of Heaven and Hell are different. I mean, they don't look like earth as we know it. Dante gave us a pretty good idea of what Hell looks like. And in Heaven we have Angels. Now, of course, Noah after the flood, started all over again with his cargo of animals. So I suppose we can take some stock in that.

LOU: I asked Fred about speeding up the returns. Because if we could, we'd get *Ubermensche*s quicker, and that would help things a lot. I used the analogy of twelve monkeys writing endlessly with pen and paper. Eventually, you'd think they could produce all the works of Shakespeare.

OVERBECK: I should imagine.

LOU: Now suppose we took away the pens from the monkeys and gave them typewriters, which operate faster. They should be able to produce at least one complete collection of all of Shakespeare in a faster time.

OVERBECK: Stands to reason.

LOU: Then, by analogy, substituting the natural forces in the universe, or the teeny weenie bits of atoms, subatoms and energy particles, for the generation of words, an *Ubermensch* could, according to Fred, produce a faster process that would, and it would diminish or shrink the times between the returns.

OVERBECK: Makes sense to me.

LOU: Let's for a moment look way into to the future. A hundred years from now. Now just suppose an *Ubermensch* came along and developed an even faster typewriter than we have today. For arguments sake, let's say one that could perform roughly 10-to-the-14th (or 100 trillion) operations per second.

OVERBECK: I'd like to be around to see that!

LOU: And to simplify matters, the *Ubermensch* puts just one monkey at the keyboard. It takes about 100 operations to generate a random character. In other words, if the monkey types a character at random, say it hits the letter "y", it will take a hundred keystrokes at random to hit that same character "y" again. Crediting today's monkey with an ability to type at 60 words per minute, that means the typewriter of the future could type about a trillion times faster. For example, while today's monkey, on average, will take about two hours to type the word "and," the *Ubermensch*s typewriter computer, on average, could manage to type the same word about 250 million times every second.

OVERBECK: I'm beginning to see why Friedrich is so attracted to you.

LOU: I estimate the complete works of Shakespeare to be 30 volumes of about 50,000 words each. The *Ubermensch*'s faster typewriter would take, on average, just shy of 10-to-the-one-millionth hours to chance upon the correct sequence. This is far more than a light year. Light, traveling at 186,000 miles per second, for a period of year, travels 5.878 trillion miles. That's 5.878 times 10 to the 12th power. So, 10-to-the-one-millionth hours is a very, very long time, wouldn't you say? By comparison, 10-to-the-64th is about the number of seconds that have elapsed since the beginning of the universe. 10-to-the-65th is ten times as big as that number, and ten-to-the-66th is a hundred times as big. 10-to-the-81st is roughly the total number of atoms that comprise the universe. 10-to-the-one-millionth, on the other hand, is so big that there is no metaphor or imaginative device that even helps to comprehend its massiveness, unless, of course, you're Mr. Friedrich Nietzsche with your fancy, schmantzy Eternal Return. One could reasonably expect the universe to implode on itself, in fact, several billion or trillion times over, before the typewriter ever types the complete works of Shakespeare. Now, one would still expect the monkey to take a trillion times longer to type the sequence, but when dealing with lengths of times this large, a trillion times faster or slower is a trivial difference. In short, while in theory both the monkey and the *Ubermensch*'s super typewriter should be able to type the complete works sooner or later, in practice it's safe to assume that neither ever will.

NIETZSCHE: *(Nietzsche rises from the bed. Raises his hand in protest.)* You miss the point, you Russian bitch demon. You monkey without breasts. *(He stumbles to the bureau.)* The two roads converge at the path. *(He retches into the wash basin.)* I can't sleep with all your infernal blabbering. *(Violently kicks over the wooden chair.)* The camel, the lion, the eagle . . . I can hardly think with all your nonstop addlepated chattering. *(Collapses back onto the bed\ and buries himself under the covers.)*

LOU: I didn't think he could hear us.

OVERBECK: Apparently he can.

LOU: And I don't care! And that's just with 26 letters in the alphabet. The molecular table, the last time I looked, had some 60 elements. So the permutations multiply even farther at the most basic of atomic levels. On a higher level, the number of species of living beings, birds, mammals, fish, amoebae, bacteria and fungi, is innumerable. You know, Professor Overbeck, I'm beginning to think that the real hitch in Mr. Friedrich Nietzsches Eternal Return is his presumption of infinity. I have to say, pardon me—but now I'm on a roll—I agree with Fred about mathematics. Is infinity a reality or a mathematical construct? The concept of infinity, mathematically speaking is based on the idea that you can always add one more. Endlessly. But does it really work in practicality? That's the fascinating thing about Zeno's famous puzzle. If you can always add one to get an infinite number, then you can always subtract or divide one to get a negative infinity. According to Zeno, if you walk toward a wall, and with each step, walk half the distance, you will never get to the wall. But go ahead and try it! You'll bump right into the wall.

OVERBECK: Dear me!

LOU: Theoretically, each of the elements in the atomic table should be endlessly divisible by half. That means that there may be things out there that even Mr. Friedrich Nietzsche doesn't know about. You have to throw them into the permutations, too, if they actually exist. Who's to say? In ancient times, there were only four elements: earth, air, water and fire. We've come a long way. And, if by a lark, some *ubermensch* finds some more elements—say like the snark that English mathematician Lewis Carroll, or O'Carroll, or whatever, wrote about—the game gets more complicated, doesn't it?

OVERBECK: If you read Genesis, the world was created in one mighty, one-time blast. Explain that.

LOU: Oh sure, we're talking about probabilistic calculations. When I say it will "on

average" take the monkey such-and-such a length of time to get a given sequence, that's the same as saying that if you play the lottery, and the odds of winning are 1 out of 50 million, then "on average" you could expect to win the lotto the fifty-millionth time you played. Of course, you could play 100 million times and still not win, or you could get lucky and win the very first time you played. In theory, the monkey could get lucky and type out the entire complete works on his first attempt. So, if Fred's actually talking about the Eternal Return of the entire universe in exact sequence, from historical geologic to geologic and historical to historical epochs, I suppose, on the off chance, it could happen, in an infinity of time. But you couldn't reasonably expect either of these things to happen. Or could you?
(Overbeck drains his glass of schnapps.)
LOU: At the bottom of it all, Fred's conclusion is that there's no birth and no death. Every moment, every person's minute-by-minute stage of life, is an infinity of energy, guided by chance and necessity. Maybe he's just a very wild poet. Or maybe the Eternal Return is Fred's way of searching for the spiritual. Maybe he's just come up with a new metaphor for the age-old metaphor for spirituality?
OVERBECK: I knew it!
LOU: Or, is he just plain nuts? Frankly, I vote for just plain nuts.
OVERBECK: No. There must be something more. The Holy Father . . .
LOU: Listen! Just consider for a moment. Friedrich makes no sense. Sure, Fred suffers. But how can he tolerate the thought of suffering millions and millions of times again? Shouldn't once be enough? I know it would be for me. The body and mind are one. Thinking and suffering are identical for Fred. Suffering. Thinking about suffering. Thinking about not suffering. Thinking about past suffering. These are his biggest joys. Honestly, Professor Overbeck, he gets off on this stuff. If he rests, recuperates, gets physically well, he gets too close to the real demon in his soul. Rest, recuperation and idleness is OK, but it's not a permanent solution. Once he gets close to equilibrium, the apple cart always tilts back to upheaval.
OVERBECK: It's the Devil in him!
LOU: Oh, please, Professor Overbeck, now you're starting to give *me* a headache. Fred is sick in a body that he doesn't think is his in which positive and negative forces are fighting. The whole thing—his pain, severe migraine headaches, fatigue, neurasthenia, nervous tension, depression, you name it—is an elaborate mental, psychological escape.
OVERBECK: Many of the Saints have experienced the same.

LOU: The more I think about it, the reason he has the world's biggest migraine headache is because he may have the world's biggest psychosis. His brain is caught in a vicious circle. The feeling of eternity and the externalization of desire are merged into a single moment. There's no before life. There's no after life. There's no beyond. It is the same. It's the same eternal life constantly, moment by moment—by the way define a moment if you will—individuated, lived and experienced throughout its individual differences. Any way you cut it, it's the same life. His. Mentally, it's the eternal return to the same old, same old. Psychologically, he wants to overcome his pain and his own self, which is the bearer of that pain. Psychologically, the *ubermensch* is a surrogate for him. He's not really talking about mankind's quest to overcome the human condition to create something new and beautiful and pure. What he's after, with all this *ubermensch* and Eternal Return nonsense is a brand new him. I mean, after all, in all honesty, who would want to be him? Not me. Not in a million years. That's for sure. Boy, is he mad!

(Nietzsche bolts upright in the bed.)

NIETZSCHE: I must confess that the deepest objection to the Eternal Recurrence is always my mother and my sister. A life with them would be an eternal hell!

(Overbeck hastens to the bedside, and pats Nietzsche on the shoulder comfortingly.)

OVERBECK: Your mother and sister are the closest thing to you. They are your blood relations. You really don't mean what you say.

NIETZSCHE: The hell I don't. Son of a bitch! One would have to go back centuries to find the noblest of races the earth has ever possessed in so instinctively pristine a degree as I present. I have, against everything that is today called *noblesse*, a sovereign feeling of distinction—I wouldn't award to the young German Kaiser the honor of being my coachman. There is one single case where I acknowledge my equal—I recognize it with profound gratitude. Frau Cosima Wagner is by far the noblest nature; and, so that I shouldn't say one word too few, I say that Richard Wagner was by far the most closely related man to me . . . The rest is silence . . . All the prevalent notions of degrees of kinship are physiological nonsense in an unsurpassable measure. The Pope still deals today in this nonsense. One is the least related to one's parents: it would be the most extreme sign of vulgarity to be related to one's parents. Higher measures have their origins infinitely farther back, and with them much had to be assembled, saved and hoarded. The great individuals are the oldest: I don't understand it, but Julius Caesar could be my father—or Alexander . . . *(Nietzsche collapses back down.)*

OVERBECK: *(To Lou.)* I always thought he was Polish? Could have fooled me there.

LOU: He's not Polish. He somehow got it in his crazy head of his that he is. Some link to some distant relation. Fred's as German as a bratwurst.

OVERBECK: *(Thoughtfully, to Lou.)* There's much to be said for stable life of routine. Family, community, country. The world is built upon it. What would life be without it?

LOU: *(Polishing her nails.)* Sure, I've got to admit that a woman likes a little stability and predictability in her life, but not the same old, same old, forever and ever, if you know what I mean. Speaking for myself, you've gotta add a little kirsch to the coffee now and then.

OVERBECK: What, do you think, causes his horrible suffering? Original sin?

LOU: Hardly. Who knows? Me? His other failed romances? A troubled childhood? And here I paraphrase from the man himself: a miscommunication between the molecules of his organic anatomy. Or any old excuse to ingest the world's largest amounts of opiates. Wow, hold it right there, talk about a vicious circle!

OVERBECK: Hey, you're right! Talk about Eternal Return! That's all he seems to do. Go at it. Recuperate. And go at it again.

LOU: Do you have any idea where he ever dreamed up this cookoo idea? This Eternal Return nonsense?

OVERBECK: As a matter of fact, yes, I do. He was at Sils-Maria recuperating. I know from his letters to me and that gossip Malwida von Meysenbug, that while the idea came to him while he was at Sils-Maria, thinking hard and intensely like no human ever has ever before. He was going through his usual attacks of intense migraines, crippling headaches, vomiting, retching, fever, debilitating fatigue, muscular paralysis, anorexia, severe constipation, heavy night sweats, hemorrhoids, eye pain, loss of eyesight, vertigo, gastric pain, stomach cramps, disequilibrium, sinking into unconsciousness . . .

LOU: Enough! I get the picture. Spare me the details.

OVERBECK: And then the idea came to him in the form of a circle in the flash of a delirious, ecstatic hallucinatory revelation.

LOU: No opiates? He was off the sauce?

OVERBECK: To the best of anyone's knowledge.

(Nietzsche gets out of bed. He strides sprightly back and forth across the room.)

NIETZSCHE: Good intestines. That's the secret. Nutriment, place and climate. I was 6,000 feet beyond man and time. Beside a mighty pyramid of rock in the woods beside the lake of Silvaplana. The salvation of mankind depends more on nutriment, climate and place than upon any quaint curiosity of the theologians. Climate influences the metabolism. The metabolism can be slow or speedy. If it's slow, man's animalistic vigor never grows sufficiently great for him to attain that freedom overflowing in the most spiritual domain he knows.

LOU: And so, I don't mean to be indiscreet, but just exactly what does that have to do with your, ah, intestines?

NIETZSCHE: I'm so glad you asked. Even so infinitesimal sluggishness of the intestines grown into a bad habit completely suffices to transform a genius into something mediocre. Something German. The German climate alone is enough to discourage strong and even heroic intestines. The tempo of the metabolism stands in exact relationship to the mobility or lameness of the feet of the spirit; the spirit itself is indeed only a species of this metabolism.

LOU: And would you care to enlighten us as to what countries or climate are most, shall we say, intestinally correct?

NIETZSCHE: Ah, give me Paris, Provence, Florence, Jerusalem, Athens. These names prove something. That genius is conditioned by dry air, clear sky—that is to say by rapid metabolism, by the possibility of again and again supplying oneself with great, even tremendous quantities of energy.

OVERBECK: While we're on the subject. I was going to ask before, but we got sidetracked, but, medically speaking, have you been regular?

NIETZSCHE: Yes, yes, my dear fellow. Ever since I stopped eating German cookery. German cookery is general—what does it not have on its conscience! Soup *before* the meal. Meat cooked to shreds, greasy and floury vegetables. The degeneration of puddings to paperweights! If one adds to this the downright bestial dinner-drinking habits of the ancient and by no means the ancient German, one will also understand the origin of the German spirit—disturbed intestines. The German spirit is an indigestion.

(Nietzsche strides off side stage.)

You must excuse me for a moment. I feel the need to commune with nature.

OVERBECK: He's certainly not going to take a walk in the woods at a time like this. He's not dressed properly.

LOU: No, Professor. I think he just went to the bathroom.

OVERBECK: Is it that he experiences his philosophy because of his body—to relieve his horrible bodily suffering? I mean, he's got nothing to fall back on for support. Unless it's drugs. And the body becomes immune to those. He has no faith. He proclaimed God dead. Religion dead. Or is it that, because he has forsaken God, religion and anything beyond, that he experiences existence in the raw, and it's this confrontation that wracks his body so? I mean, after all, the mind and the body are one. Not separate and indivisible like some would have you think, like that damn Frenchman Descartes. What's doing the suffering here? The mind or the body? When I come to think of it, Friedrich, with all his intense and horrible suffering, might actually be quite a happy man. He overcomes his suffering with the vision of the *uberniensch* so he can create his great works.

(Nietzsche returns. He stands at the end of the stage listening.)

LOU: Or maybe, just maybe, he's just got a headache. After all, we all get them now and then. And, maybe, just coincidentally, he just happens to be thinking about these things at the same time. I once asked Paul about the origin of migraine, when he Fred and I were palling around together. Every doctor agrees that the blood vessels, particularly the temporal arteries, have a role in a migraine attack. The vessels constrict and then engorge. The pain may come from the constricted vessels themselves, or from the organs which need their normal blood supply and find it impeded, especially brain membranes.

OVERBECK: But why do the blood vessels constrict?

LOU: That's a very good question. Nobody seems to really know. There's only specu-lation. Some physicians think that there's an underlying pathology of migraine. A rhythm disorder—a biochemical, social-psychological or stress disorder. They seem to think the rhythm disorder is more important than the headache itself.

OVERBECK: I'm afraid I don't understand what you're saying.

LOU: By rhythm disorder, I believe what they're saying is that there's a disequi-librium in the normal rhythms of the psyche or consciousness or life styles or experiences of the individual.

OVERBECK: You mean their lives are screwed up?

LOU: Yes. Something in their lives has caused an imbalance of their basic psychic energies. It expresses itself in physical symptoms. Their bodies are telling them there's something wrong in their lives, their relationships, their thinking, their environment, the way they behave. The body and the brain do not work alone.

OVERBECK: If I follow you, this would mean that the emotions and the mind have a direct affect [*sic*] on the physical body. This is very unorthodox. It circumvents the soul, God's role and the place of the priest.

LOU: Professor Overbeck, I like you a lot, but let's not go overboard. Let's stick to the issue at hand. Some doctors say the rhythm disorder may express itself in vari-ous ways. They say some patients say they have a sharp pain in their side or above their elbow, or a crippling soreness in their leg. But when the doctor investigates, there's nothing there physically to be found. No trauma, no tumor, no laceration, lesion, cut, bruise or injury. It's pain without a physical cause. The disequilibrium of the psyche can express itself through any number of organs. Thus, the headache itself need not be present in an attack of so-called migraine. There may be sharp attacks of stomach pain, as opposed to head pain.

OVERBECK: Like suddenly getting sick in the stomach over something or some event.

LOU: Yes, exactly. Or suddenly getting an erection over a beautiful woman.

OVERBECK: *(Fidgets nervously.)* I wouldn't know anything about that.

LOU: *(Stares at Overbeck sarcastically?)* No, of course, not. Come to think of it, I don't know where his schwanz has been since we broke up. But there's also some reason to believe that migraine headaches of Friedrich's severity could be caused by venereal disease.

(Nietzsche steps forward.)

NIETZSCHE: Oh, *Hetaera esmeralda*. Oh, Esmeralda, your powdered demiglobes in a Spanish bodice, your nut brown skin and black hair. What I wouldn't give for one more night in Graz. To recklessly tempt fate. To spurn salvation and receive the demonic. Yes, I would do it again.

LOU: I don't care in the least to hear about your past affairs, Fred. Can't you think of something else to talk about?

NIETZSCHE: I am a disciple of the philosopher Dionysus. I'd rather be a satyr than a saint.

LOU: But tell me, though. This Esmeralda creature. Was this before or after me?

NIETZSCHE: Before. Way before I knew you.

LOU: And?

NIETZSCHE: I do not object to a man who takes sex when he needs it. But I hate the man who begs for it, who gives up *his* power to the dispensing woman. To the crafty woman who turns *her* weakness, and *his* strength, into *her* strength. When you go to women, don't forget your whip!

LOU: *(Glares at Nietzsche. Then turns to Overbeck.)* Would you care for another schnapps, Professor Overbeck? Actually, if we're going to have another glass, may I drop the formal and address you in the second person informal? After all, Franz, we've known each other for twenty years.

OVERBECK: I don't see why not. But no, thank you, enough schnapps for me. Too much schnapps puts me on edge.

LOU: Well, good. There's just enough for one more. *(She pours the remainder of the schnapps bottle into her glass.)* You don't mind?

OVERBECK: Not at all. *(Looks about the room.)* But, I was wondering, though, might there be a little weed on the premises?

LOU: Oh, Fred's got everything.

OVERBECK: *(Assays the bottle-laden bureau top):* Hmm. You know, I'm not used to all this heavy, constant philosophizing. Quiet old churches and country graveyards are my thing. Forget the weed. I wonder, if, just by chance, there just may be some opium in this household pharmacy? To clear my head, of course.

(Nietzsche tosses and turns on the bed. He puts a pillow over his head.)

LOU: *(Yells across the room.)* Hey, Fred, which one's the opium?

NIETZSCHE: *(Yells back in great distress.)* The green bottle!

OVERBECK: *(Picks up a bottle.)* This says laudanum.

NIETZSCHE: No, no. The one next to it. In the second row.

OVERBECK: Oh, this little brown bottle. No that's not it. It's marked codeine.

NIETZSCHE: No, you idiot. Can't you see? Where are your eyes? It's right in front of you, in the back. Right next to the chloral. Do I, who can barely walk, whose head is splitting, have to get out of bed and show you! *(Grasps his head.)* Ohhh, ohhhh, ohhh!

OVERBECK: Ah, yes. Here it is. *(Picks up a bottle and takes a long draught from it.)* Ahhh. God is that good!

NIETZSCHE: How many times have I told you not to mention that word ever again in this house!

LOU: He only meant it as a figure of speech.

NIETZSCHE: That's the whole problem with civilization. Figures of speech. We say things we don't even know the meaning of. "I await you with bated breath." "You're goldbricking?" "Never stare a gift horse in the mouth." "A bellwether sign." We just say them because we've always said them. Most of the time, we don't know what they mean. What's a bated breath? What does a gold brick have to do with indolence? Why am I "pleased as Punch"? What's the matter with looking in a horse's mouth? Who knows? Who cares? What does a castrated sheep have to do with anything? "My goose is cooked." I don't even own a goose. And, if I did want it cooked, would I want it medium, rare or well done? Just what is a "month of Sundays?" Why not a month of Saturdays? Can't you, for once, be a little more creative, a little more unique, just a bit more original?

LOU: Oh, and I suppose the *Ubermensch* could say it better?

NIETZSCHE: Yes.

LOU: Like?

NIETZSCHE: Like . . . like . . . this opiate has swept away the dark clouds that separate my conscious mind from my unconscious. Or, this tincture of ambrosial delight has sent my senses reeling beyond the confines of earthly concerns; I kick my heels and dance, yes, dance, in joy with the stars, with the celestial seraphim of the great unknowable beyond. *(Grasps his head.)* Ohhhh! Ohhh! Ohhh! My head. My head.

LOU: Now what's the matter?

NIETZSCHE: I did it to myself. Didn't you hear? Seraphim. A figure of speech. I only meant it poetically. But worse yet. An old ecclesiastical word, concept. My work is so daunting. I don't know if I'm up to the task. I don't know if any human is up the task. It will take many generations of overmen to override this curse. Curse? What curse? From where? Whose curse? *(Grasps his head.)* Ohhh! Ohhh! Ohhh! My head, my head, my poor, tormented head. There I go, I've done it again.

OVERBECK: (To Lou.) I've got to go. I'll miss my train.

LOU: I'll go with you. There's not much I can do here.

OVERBECK: He's all alone.

LOU: He's always been alone. He does it to himself.

OVERBECK: Yes, maybe you're right. But he's always gotten through these torments, these hours of delirium and suffering. And, I suppose, in the end, he's always got his sister.

LOU: That bitch!

OVERBECK: Now, now. You may not like her. But she's always been there for him. Maybe if he had a pet, it would ease his loneliness. A dog, perhaps.

LOU: A dog requires care. It has to be taken on walks.

OVERBECK: Well, yes. Perhaps a cat.

LOU: Cats need feeding, care and affection.

OVERBECK: Hmm. Maybe a bird. Say, a parrot? *(Lou glares at him in amazement.)* Yes, quite right. Forget it. Imagine that!

LOU: Your train.

OVERBECK: Oh yes. We've got to be going, Friedrich. Please get some rest. Some sleep.

NIETZSCHE: Goodbye, Overbeck.

LOU: Goodbye, Fred. We may see one another, again. But I wouldn't hold your breath, if I were you.

NIETZSCHE: I am the anti-Christ!

LOU: And I am the Empress Napoleon.

NIETZSCHE: Auf weidersein, mein little, sweet pickled herring. Mein liebchen.

LOU: Fred, get a life!

(Lou and Overbeck exit.)

NIETZSCHE: *(Forlorn.)* Well, here I am, again, all alone. Nobody but me and my headache. What would I do without you, where would I be without you headache, my old friend? Yes, just me and my headache. *(Pauses.)* Headache . . . *(Drags himself to the bureau. Pours draughts of liquid into a glass, and swallows deeply. Stiffens upright. His body convulses.)* Yes, my headache, my headache, my dear, dear headache . . . *(He turns and dances the soft-shoe. Smoke rises about him. He grows taller.)* And the Will to Power! *(He dances.)* Whatever does not kill me, makes me stronger!

NIETZSCHE: *(Waves to the audience. The music of Wagner's "Ride of the Valkeryies" with a Disney, Loony Tunes-cartoon tempo, starts.)* That's all, folks. See you later!

(As the curtain descends, a big, pink bunny, like the Energizer Bunny, mechanically walks the length of the stage in front of the curtain beating a big bass drum upon which is emblazoned: "Eternal Return.")

CURTAIN

(In the lobby, by the doors, as the audience leaves, stand several actors who are exact replicas of Nietszche.)

ACTOR(S): Thanks for coming! Come again!

THE END

Hoofbeats in the Head

EDWARD LOWBURY

Hoofbeats in the head—the nightmare's return
With a flurry of sparks, a cloud of graveyard thoughts;
The mind shrinks from a blank cemetery of noughts
And crosses. People watch, but it's not their concern.
You are wide awake, and still the dream goes on; the hooves
Have followed you from sleep. It's day, and yet the light
Stays hidden . . . Now for sharper eyes to recover sight,
And power to beat the beast in a few simple moves!

I Know Upon Awakening

KATHLEEN J. O'SHEA

I lift my head gingerly off the pillow this morning, and every morning, to know what kind of day I will live. When I awake with a full-blown attack, it's often too late to "rescue" the force of the event I will face. If I lift my head and find it heavy to hold up, with that all-too-familiar deep pain in the right side of my neck, along the occipital nerve, my fate for the earlier future is still up in the air.

Sometimes I can stop it—that is if I can function well enough to break the glass vial, open the packages of syringe and filter needle, fill the syringe with the DHE, change back the end of the syringe from the filter to the needle, and give myself an injection in my thigh. If I can think clearly enough to remember the anti-nausea medicine, I may be spared an additional agony.

If the pain moves to a throbbing, pounding pain behind my right eye, I haven't caught it in time, and the nausea and vomiting are much more agonizing, trying to survive, having my head and arms lying on the toilet seat as I try to vomit away the nausea. Migraine has now taken ownership of my body and my psyche.

Another distinct possibility is that what I'll carry with me this day, and likely several more, is extreme tightness in the right side of my neck, with pain so great in this one tiny spot deep in the muscles along the occipital nerve, I long for someone or something to bear down there with as much pressure as possible. The trigger points at the base of my skull feel like swollen knots, very tender to the touch. This day will be, with luck, "just" a functional day, one where I can carry on with only the skeleton of living.

These are the "functional" days, when I also carry the other, sometimes "invisible" parts of living with migraine: cognitive, memory, and psychological effects. My headache specialist, Dr. Joseph Mann, once suggested the analogy that if my head were a computer, what it needs is to be rebooted, and that's what it feels like; something just feels wrong in the brain. Sometimes, I even feel what seem to be electrical currents going haywire.

Often, I draw blanks mid-sentence, lose names of things or people, forget something someone just told me, move clumsily, and am weak and weary. I cry easily, fight irritability and mood swings, live with digestive problems, and if the days turn into weeks or, just recently, months, I start to carry guilt for affecting my loved ones and friends.

What if it never "breaks" this time? This fear and living with the constant threat that one wrong turn of my neck will throw me into the wrenching pain of a full-blown headache leave me very anxious. The awful truth is that many of my symptoms, when in a "functional" stage, I can hide from all but close friends and family, but the hiding is such a struggle and further supports the opinion of so many that "It's just a headache." Much of migraine is invisible to most and lonely for the migraineur.

What's not invisible is the ecstasy of waking up and knowing right away that the migraine cycle has broken; I lift my head on these days feeling like a real force has moved out of my brain and body; suddenly, I'm me again. Do some people wake up this way most days? I never have more gratitude and mindfulness than I do when I experience this "lift." I pay attention to all the beauty of the day, and I have energy because now I can live rather than exist—at least for this moment.

But, migraine waits for me. What if I try to do too much? What if it comes back? No, *when* will it come back? A turn of the head, a jarring movement, a time of stress, staring into the computer screen too long. Chronic migraineurs live with this fear.

I want to learn to live with migraine as the disease that it is, accepting that it is not separate from me but really a part of who I am. It's a struggle, though. My life with migraine began when I was 14, moved from episodic migraine to chronic migraine in my 30's, and has had its peaks and valleys ever since. For years I was blessed with a compassionate and persistent team of doctors, many of whom have been with me on this journey for years as well as a patient, loving support system of family and friends. While I have more bad days than good, I appreciate the good ones more than someone without migraine; the sun is brighter, the smells are richer, the air is fresher.

PART III

It's Just a Headache?

Introduction

People with migraine not only contend with the invisibility of their condition but mercilessly cope with the underestimation of the disease, the idea that "it's just a headache." Migraineurs do not yet live in a society able to empathize with this multidimensional disease. Part III hopes to enlighten varied audiences about migraine, a disease that takes center stage in a person's life. While so many people ask about "the headache," the person with migraine knows that the effects are on the whole self. For the migraine sufferer, migraine is not just an aspect of her life she must deal with. There is no other self not experiencing the migraine: A noncomprehending observer may not understand this.

Oliver Sacks in "A General Feeling of Disorder" argues,

> Though there are many (one is tempted to say, innumerable) possible presentations of common migraine—I described nearly a hundred such in my book—its commonest harbinger may be just an indefinable but undeniable feeling of *something amiss*. This is exactly what Emil du Bois-Reymond emphasized when, in 1860, he described his own attacks of migraine: "I wake," he writes, "with a general feeling of disorder...."[1]

Most people we know still use the terms "migraine" and "headache" interchangeably. Often a well-intentioned acquaintance or friend frequently offers, "I get migraines, too; do you want a couple of Advil ... You can't go out *again* tonight; you're going to let a headache get in the way of this night we planned a week ago ... You don't look sick; you looked fine an hour ago ... have you tried ..." Migraineurs have heard these pronouncements and others—all reminders that this remains a disease largely misunderstood in terms of its debilitation and complexity. These (and many more) common responses to migraine can make the sufferer so much more lonely and mislabeled.

Friends, employers, coworkers, and medical professionals might grasp in these readings some of the more common adjacent symptoms to the headache—hypersensitivity to touch, light, and sound; severe neck pain; an overwhelming draining of energy, where every step seems hard; as well as psychological effects, including mood swings, anxiety, and depression, as we see with Anita Brookner's protagonist in her novel *A Misalliance*:

> The headache had settled down to a heaviness in the eyes and a sensitivity in the skin of the face and the head; she would be unable to brush her hair for another night. Lying in bed was all that she was required to do, but now she felt less comfortable about it. The sadness of childhood recalled, and the greater sadness that had come with her middle age, turned her thoughts to melancholy and the desire for consolation.[2]

In the poem "Six Explanations for Migraine," by Lisa Guskin-Stonestreet, the persona struggles with how to explain this overwhelming force that she lives with, as well as all of its manifestations:

> *If the affection be protracted, the patient*
> *will die; if more light*
>
> *and not deadly it becomes chronic, torpor*
> *and weariness.* Cold cloths,
>
> supplications. Offerings
> to the gods. *Sharp and tormenting*
>
> *Vapors.* Pull the drapes, safe
> from sight. Dim
>
> the light, damp half
> the mind, and wait.[3]

Other fiction writers, including Irvin Yalom and Tobias Wolff, speak to the loneliness that comes from the all-consuming pain and illness. Many days, one must use every bit of concentration and energy to cope with all that constitutes migraine, and, yet, "it's just a headache" to most of the people we encounter in our daily lives: "she despised the self-pitying tone of the newsletter, and its spurious implication that readers were not alone in their suffering. Because they were alone. In fact everyone was alone all the time, but when you got sick you knew it, and that is a lot of what suffering was—knowing."[4]

The female chronic migraineur also must even sometimes sacrifice the fundamental role of parenting. This sacrifice is one that obviously, too, extends to her partner. Not only does she sometimes question her ability to adequately parent a child when so much of her life is consumed by this disease, but she must recognize that during pregnancy she will undoubtedly have to stop taking important medications that she needs to prevent acute attacks of migraine. In an excerpt from the novel *Claire's Head* (a scene not included in this anthology), the protagonist struggles to help her husband understand why she's reluctant to have a baby.

It's not surprising that a partner in a relationship should sometimes be impatient and see only the disruption in the present moment. Dina, Joyce's partner in Wolff's "Migraine," says irritably to Joyce, "I can't plan a trip to the beach without you pulling this stuff."[5]

Again, what the observer—whether it's a partner, a friend, or even a doctor—can fail to recognize are the fear, guilt, and anxiety the sufferer lives with on a regular basis, often worrying about making commitments, promises, and plans. This realization along with the other facets of migraine disease are important for the migraineur and others to understand and communicate; these are very real components of migraine, ones that separate it from the occasional or even frequent headache.

NOTES

1. Oliver Sacks, *Hallucinations* (New York: Penguin Random House, 2012), 168–69 (emphasis added).
2. Anita Brookner, *A Misalliance* (New York: Vintage Books, 2005), 171.
3. Lisa Gluskin-Stonestreet, "Six Explanations of Migraine," *Blackbird* 14, no. 1 (2015): lines 11–20, https://blackbird.vcu.edu/v14n1/poetry/stonestreet_1 /migraine_page.shtml.
4. Tobias Wolff, "Migraine," in *The Night in Question* (New York: Vintage Books, 1996), 173.
5. Wolff, "Migraine," 179.

A General Feeling of Disorder

OLIVER SACKS

No one has written more eloquently about [the need for harmony with the two divisions of the autonomic nervous system in order to feel "well"] than Antonio Damasio in his book *The Feeling of What Happens* and many subsequent books and papers. He speaks of a "core consciousness," the basic feeling of *how one is,* which eventually becomes a dim, implicit feeling of consciousness. It is especially when things are going wrong, internally—when homeostasis is not being maintained; when the autonomic balance starts listing heavily to one side or the other—that this core consciousness, the feeling of how one is, takes on an intrusive, unpleasant quality, and now one will say, "I feel ill—something is amiss." At such times one no longer looks well either.

As an example of this, migraine is a sort of prototype illness, often very unpleasant but transient, and self-limiting; benign in the sense that it does not cause death or serious injury and that it is not associated with any tissue damage or trauma or infection; and occurring only as an often-hereditary disturbance of the nervous system. Migraine provides, in miniature, the essential features of being ill—of trouble inside the body—without actual illness.

When I came to New York, nearly fifty years ago, the first patients I saw suffered from attacks of migraine—"common migraine," so called because it attacks at least 10 percent of the population. (I myself have had attacks of them throughout my life.) Seeing such patients, trying to understand or help them, constituted my apprenticeship in medicine—and led to my first book, *Migraine*.

Though there are many (one is tempted to say, innumerable) possible presentations of common migraine—I described nearly a hundred such in my book—its commonest harbinger may be just an indefinable but undeniable feeling of something amiss. This is exactly what Emil du Bois-Reymond emphasized when, in 1860, he described his own attacks of migraine: "I wake," he writes, "with a general feeling of disorder. . . ."

In his case (he had had migraines every three to four weeks, since his twentieth year), there would be "a slight pain in the region of the right temple which . . . reaches its greatest intensity at midday; towards evening it usually passes off. . . . At rest the pain is bearable, but it is increased by motion to a high degree of violence. . . . It responds to each beat of the temporal artery." Moreover, du Bois-Reymond looked different during his migraines: "The countenance is pale and sunken, the right eye small and reddened." During violent attacks he would experience nausea and "gastric disorder." The "general feeling of disorder" that so often inaugurates migraines may continue, getting more and more severe in the course of an attack; the worst-affected patients may be reduced to lying in a leaden haze, feeling half-dead, or even that death would be preferable.

I cite du Bois-Reymond's self-description, as I do at the very beginning of *Migraine,* partly for its precision and beauty (as are common in nineteenth-century neurological descriptions, but rare now), but above all, because it is *exemplary*—all cases of migraine vary, but they are, so to speak, permutations of his.

The vascular and visceral symptoms of migraine are typical of unbridled para-sympathetic activity, but they may be preceded by a physiologically opposite state. One may feel full of energy, even a sort of euphoria, for a few hours before a migraine—George Eliot would speak of herself as feeling "dangerously well" at such times. There may, similarly, especially if the suffering has been very intense, be a "rebound" *after* a migraine. This was very clear with one of my patients (Case #68 in *Migraine*), a young mathematician with very severe migraines. For him the resolution of a migraine, accompanied by a huge passage of pale urine, was always followed by a burst of original mathematical thinking. "Curing" his migraines, we found, "cured" his mathematical creativity, and he elected, given this strange economy of body and mind, to keep both.

While this is the general pattern of a migraine, there can occur rapidly changing fluctuations and contradictory symptoms—a feeling that patients often call "unsettled." In this unsettled state (I wrote in *Migraine*), "one may feel hot or cold, or both . . . bloated and tight, or loose and queasy; a peculiar tension, or languor, or both . . . sundry strains and discomforts, which come and go."

Indeed, everything comes and goes, and if one could take a scan or inner photograph of the body at such times, one would see vascular beds opening and closing, peristalsis accelerating or stopping, viscera squirming or tightening in spasms, secretions suddenly increasing or decreasing—as if the nervous system itself were in a state of indecision. Instability, fluctuation, and oscillation are of the essence in the unsettled state, this general feeling of disorder. We lose the normal feeling of "wellness," which all of us, and perhaps all animals, have in health.

Migraine

TOBIAS WOLFF

It began while she was at work. At the first pang her breath caught and her eyes went wide open. Then it subsided, leaving a faint pressure at the back of her neck. Joyce put her hands on either side of the keyboard and waited. From the cubicles around her she heard the steady click of other keyboards. She knew what was happening to her, knew so well that when the next wave came she felt it not as pain but as dread for what was still to come. Joyce closed down the terminal, then gathered the lab reports and put them in a folder.

She stopped in the doorway of her supervisor's office to say that she was leaving early. Her supervisor made a sympathetic face and offered to call a cab if Joyce didn't feel up to the drive; she could pay for it out of petty cash. "That's what it's there for," she said.

"I'll manage," Joyce told her. She added: "You don't have to whisper."

Joyce did not drive home. Instead she called a taxi from the lobby of the building, as she had intended to do all along. Her supervisor might think that she was giving the money freely, but it wouldn't work out that way. Whatever people gave you from their overflowing hearts they remembered, and expected you to remember, forever. In Joyce's experience there was no such thing as petty cash.

When she got home she found two cardboard boxes in the living room, filled with her roommate's few belongings. Joyce and Dina had quarreled again, and now Dina was taking the final step in their agreement that she should move out. Joyce looked at the boxes. She considered searching through them, then rejected the idea as beneath her. It was the kind of thing she used to do but had taught herself, with difficulty, to stop doing. She closed her eyes for a moment, swaying slightly from side to side, then crossed the room and turned the television on. A screaming host in a yellow blazer was trying to make himself heard over the delirium of his audience as a big clock ticked away the seconds. Joyce turned the volume off and went into the kitchen to boil some water for tea.

The newspaper was strewn over the countertop, its edges fluttering in the breeze. Dina had left the window open again. Though Joyce kept after her, she refused to take ordinary precautions and shrugged off her carelessness as the unimportant, even lovable consequence of being a free spirit with no material hang-ups. But Joyce saw through her; she understood that by playing this part Dina had forced the opposite role on her, that of the grasping neurotic. Joyce caught herself acting like this sometimes. But not anymore. All that was over now.

Joyce started the water and went to the window. She rested her elbows on the sill and held her face in her hands, kneading her temples with her fingertips. She pressed harder and harder as the pulse quickened. At the worst moment she went suddenly deaf, as if someone had pushed her head underwater. Then it passed. Joyce heard her own ragged breathing. She heard the scrabble of pigeons' feet on the tile roof and children's voices from the playground of a nearby school, a jackhammer far enough away that its sound was bearable, even companionable, like the distant sound of marching bands in the college town where she had grown up.

Joyce let the breeze cool the sweat from her face. Then she closed the window and began to fill her brewing spoon with chamomile, tilia, and spearmint.

Joyce's eyes were scratchy. Her skin felt damp, and her blouse clung coldly where it had soaked through. She carried the tea to her bedroom and left it steeping on the nightstand while she undressed and sat on the edge of her bed. The room was a mess. Clothes everywhere, hanging from hooks and knobs and bunched on the floor. Newspapers. Suitcases still packed for a visit to Dina's parents, which they'd never made because Joyce got sick. She bent to pick up a shoe, then dropped it and rocked forward onto her feet. She wrapped herself in a terry bathrobe and went to the living room, where, propped up on the sofa, she sipped her tea and watched the silent television.

The tea helped. Not much, really, but it gave Joyce the only influence she had over what was happening to her. Except for Dina's massages, nothing else worked at all. Joyce had taken medicinal baths. She'd gotten drunk and she'd gotten stoned. She had tried every remedy she'd ever heard of, barring the obviously useless ones like breathing through a scuba diver's tank. That suggestion appeared in a newsletter Dina had forced her to subscribe to until Joyce decided that reading about the problem all the time was making it worse instead of better. Also she despised the self-pitying tone of the newsletter, and its spurious implication that readers were not alone in their suffering.

Because they were alone. In fact everyone was alone all the time, but when you got sick you knew it, and that was a lot of what suffering was—knowing.

Joyce drank off the last of her tea. She set the mug down on the floor and stared at Dina's boxes. Almadén: Dina must have brought them from the liquor store. The tops were open. A white mohair sweater lay on top of one box, a jumble of bottles and tubes on top of the other. Joyce leaned back. Even with her eyes closed she could sense the flickering of the television as the camera jumped from host to contestants, contestants to host. The apartment was profoundly quiet.

It was good to be alone. Really alone, without other people around to let you imagine that your life had mingled with theirs. That never was true. Even together, people were as solitary as cows in a field chewing their own cud.

You couldn't enter the life of another person even when you wanted to. Back in August Joyce and Dina had a friend over for dinner, and in the course of the evening she told a story about a couple they all knew who'd recently been injured in a peculiar accident. A waterbed with a fat guy on it had crashed through their ceiling while they were watching TV and landed right on top of them. It was a miracle they weren't killed—not that this view of the episode would comfort them much, considering the hurts they did end up with: a broken collarbone for one, a sprained neck and concussion for the other. Joyce and Dina shook their heads when their friend came to the end of this story. They looked down at their plates. Joyce managed to keep her jaw clenched until Dina began snorting, and then all three of them let go. They howled. They couldn't stop. Joyce got so short of breath she had to push her chair back and lower her head between her knees.

And yet she had known these women. Their pain should have meant something to her. But even now, in pain herself, she couldn't feel theirs, or come any closer than thinking that she ought to feel it. And the same would be true if the waterbed had fallen on her and Dina instead of on them. Even if it had killed her they would have laughed, then afterward regretted their laughter as she had regretted hers. They'd have gone on about their business, remembering her less and less often, and always with a sudden helpless smile like the one she felt on her own lips right now.

The effects of the tea were wearing off. Joyce raised her head from the pillows and slowly sat up. She stared at the boxes again, then looked at the television. A man was smiling steadfastly while the woman next to him emptied a container of white goo over his head.

Joyce pushed herself up. She went to the kitchen and filled the kettle with fresh water, then leaned against the counter. The pulse was getting stronger again; each time it struck she dipped her head slightly, as if she were nodding off. She entered another period of deafness. When she came out of it the kettle-top was rattling; beads of water rolled down the sides, hissing against the burner. Joyce refilled the brewing spoon, poured water into her cup, and carried it back to the living room. She knelt between Dina's boxes and began searching through the one with the sweater on top.

Beneath the sweater were some photographs that Dina had kept in her vanity mirror, stuck between the glass and the frame. A whole series of her brother and his family, the two daughters getting taller from picture to picture, their sweet round faces growing thin and wary. A formal portrait of Dina's parents. Several snapshots of Joyce. Joyce glanced through these pictures and put them aside. She sat back on her heels. She drew a deep, purposeful breath and held her head erect, the very picture of a woman who has just managed to get the better of herself after a moment's weakness. The refrigerator motor kicked on. Joyce could hear bottles tinkling against each other. Joyce took another breath, then leaned forward again and continued to unpack the box.

Clothes. Shoes. A blow-dryer. Finally, at the bottom, Dina's books: *Chariots of the Gods, The Inner Game of Tennis, Many Mansions, In Search of Bigfoot, The No-Sweat Workout,* and *The Bhagavad-Gita.* Joyce opened *In Search of Bigfoot* and flipped through the illustrations. These included a voicegraph taken from a hidden microphone, the plaster cast of a large foot with surprisingly thin, fingerlike toes, and a blurry picture of the monster itself walking across a clearing with its arms swinging casually at its sides. Joyce repacked the box. No wonder her brain was eroding. Dina had so much junk in her head that just having a conversation with her was like being sandblasted.

Once Dina moved out, Joyce was going to get her mind back in shape. She had a list of books she intended to read. She was going to keep a journal and take some night classes in philosophy. Joyce had done well in her philosophy survey course back in college, so well that when her professor returned the final paper he attached a note of thanks to Joyce for helping to make the class such a pleasure to teach.

Not that Joyce thought of becoming a professional philosopher. But she felt alive when she talked about ideas, and she still remembered the calm certainty with which her professor stalked the beliefs of his students down to their origins in superstition and hearsay and mere emotion. He was famous for making people cry. Joyce became adept at this kind of argument herself. She had moments of the purest clarity when she could feel herself striking closer and closer to the truth, while observing with amused detachment the panic of some classmate in danger of forfeiting an illusion. Joyce had not felt so clear about anything since, because she had been involved with other people, and other people muddied the water. What with their needs and their demands and their feelings, their almighty anxieties to be tended to eight or nine times a day, you ended up telling so many lies that in time you forgot what the truth sounded like. But Joyce wasn't that far gone—not yet. Alone, she could begin to read again, to think, to see things as they were. Alone, she could be as cold and hard as the truth demanded. No more false cheer. No pretense of intimacy. No lies.

Another thing. No more TV. Joyce had bought it only as a way of keeping Dina quiet, but that would no longer be necessary. She picked up the remote control, watched the rest of a commercial for pickup trucks, then turned the set off. The blank screen made her uncomfortable. Jumpy, almost as if it were watching her. Joyce put the remote control back on the coffee table and began to unpack the other box.

Halfway down, between two towels, she found what she was looking for. A pair of scissors, fine German scissors that belonged to her. Joyce hadn't known she was looking for them, but when her fingers touched the blades she almost laughed out loud. Dina had taken her scissors. Deliberately. There was no chance of a mistake, because these scissors were unique. They had cunning brass handles that formed the outline of a duck's head when closed, and the blades were engraved with German words that meant "For my dear Karin from her loving father." Joyce had found the scissors at an antique store on Post Street, and from the moment she brought them home Dina had been fascinated by them. She borrowed them so often that Joyce suspected her of inventing work just to have an excuse to use them. And now she'd stolen them. Joyce held the scissors above the box and snicked them open and shut several times. Wasn't this an eye-opener, though. Little Miss Free Spirit, Miss Unencumbered by Worldly Goods would rather steal than live without a pair of scissors. She was a thief—a hypocrite and a thief.

Joyce put the scissors down beside the remote control. She pushed the heel of her hand hard against her forehead. For the first time that day she felt tired. With luck she might even be able to sleep for a while.

Joyce slid the scissors back between the towels and repacked the box. Dina could have them. There was no point in saying anything to her—she'd only feign surprise and say it was an accident—and no way for Joyce to mention the scissors without revealing that she had searched the boxes. Dina could keep the damn things, and as time went by it would begin to dawn on her, so many months, so many years later, that Joyce must know she'd stolen them; but still Joyce would not mention them, not in her Christmas cards or the friendly calls she'd make on Dina's birthday or the postcards she'd send from the various countries she planned to visit. In the end Dina would know that Joyce had pardoned her and made a gift of the scissors, and then, for the first time, she would begin to understand the kind of person Joyce really was, and how wrong she had been about her—how blind and unfeeling. At last she would know what she had lost.

When Joyce woke up, Dina was standing beside the sofa looking down at her. A few bars of pale light lay across the rug and the wall; the rest of the room was in shadow. Joyce tried to raise her head. It felt like a stone. She settled back again.

"I knew it," Dina said.

Joyce waited. When Dina just kept looking at her, she asked, "Knew what?"

"Guess." Dina turned away and went into the kitchen.

Joyce heard her running water into the kettle. Joyce called, "Are you referring to the fact that I'm sick?"

Dina didn't answer.

"It doesn't concern you," Joyce said.

Dina came to the kitchen door. "Don't do this, Joyce. At least be honest about what's happening, okay?"

"Pretend I'm not here," Joyce said. "This has nothing to do with you."

Dina shook her head. "I just can't believe you're doing this." She went back in the kitchen.

"Doing *what?*" Joyce asked. "I'm lying here on the couch. Is that what I'm doing?"

"You know," Dina said. She leaned into the doorway again and said, "Stop playing head games."

"Head games," Joyce repeated. "Jesus Mary and Joseph."

Dina took a step into the living room. "It isn't fair, Joyce."

Joyce turned onto her side. She lay motionless, listening to Dina bang around in the kitchen.

I'm not stupid!" Dina yelled.

"Nobody said you were."

Dina came into the living room carrying two cups. She set one down on the coffee table where Joyce could reach it and carried the other to the easy chair.

"Thanks," Joyce said. She sat up slowly, nodding with dizziness. She picked up the tea and held it against her chest, letting the fragrant steam warm her face.

Dina leaned forward and blew into her cup. "You look horrible," she said. Joyce smiled.

The two of them drank their tea, watching each other over the cups. "I'm going crazy," Dina said. "I can't plan a trip to the beach without you pulling this stuff."

"Ignore me," Joyce told her.

"That's what you always say. I'm leaving, Joyce. Maybe not now, but someday."

"Leave now," Joyce said.

"Do you really want me to?"

"If you're going to leave, leave now."

"You look just awful. It really hurts, doesn't it?"

"Pretend I'm not here," Joyce said.

"But I *can't.* You know I can't. That's what's so unfair. I can't just walk out when you're hurting like this."

"Dina."

"What?"

Joyce shook her head. "Nothing. Nothing."

Dina said, "Damn you, Joyce."

"You should leave," Joyce said.

"I'm going to. That's a promise. Don't ever say you didn't have fair warning."

Joyce nodded.

Dina stood and picked up one of the boxes. "I heard a great Polack joke today."

"Not now," Joyce said. "It would kill me."

Dina carried the box to her bedroom and came back for the other one, the one with the scissors. It was bulkier than the first and she had trouble getting a grip on it. "Damn you," she said to Joyce. "I can't believe I'm doing this."

Joyce finished her tea. She crossed her arms and leaned forward until her head was almost touching her knees. From Dina's bedroom she could hear the sound of drawers being yanked open and slammed shut. Then there was silence, and when Joyce raised her head Dina was standing over her again.

"Poor old Joyce," she said.

Joyce shrugged.

"Move over," Dina said. She arranged herself at the end of the sofa and said, "Okay." Joyce lay down again, her head in Dina's lap. Dina looked down at her. She brushed back a lock of Joyce's hair.

"Head games," Joyce said, and laughed.

"Shut up," Dina said.

Six Explanations for Migraine

LISA GLUSKIN-STONESTREET

1 Demon
Flashing like lightning it is loosed
above and below. Weather, wind

enters through the eye, row
of trees along the road. *Like one*

sick of heart he staggers, like one
bereft of reason he is broken.

The dance stop-
gap, hypnotic. Slips in

past the interim, ducks
through a hole in the sight.

2 Hemicrania
If the affection be protracted, the patient
will die; if more light

and not deadly it becomes chronic, torpor
and weariness. Cold cloths,

supplications. Offerings
to the gods. *Sharp and tormenting*

Vapors. Pull the drapes, safe
from sight. Dim

the light, damp half
the mind, and wait.

3 Deity
The fiery life of divine essence
aflame beyond the beauty of the meadows:

I gleam in the waters and I burn
in the sun, moon, and stars.

The world hums
in outline, glow: what he'll come

to call "the visuals"
radiating, eyebrow out.

From the very day of her birth, this woman
has lived as if caught in a net.

And I would call it down, pull out
my own shoddy wiring,

make trade of music
for this passed-on spell.

4 Psyche
Outlet for unacceptable impulses.
Harmful manifestations

of harmful processes.
Children don't—The flip

of my grandmother's skirt,
doctor's door

slamming in her wake.
Children don't: She was right,

knew the tripwire
from the cause. Still

here is a box,
a nest of wires.

Gloves, clippers. I strip
the sheath. White matter,

shutter. Know more, but still
they twist, they ghost.

Gift him the case
along with the tools.

5 Chemistry
Ibuprofen, caffeine.
Ergotamine tartrate.

Propoxyphene. Dextro-
propoxyphene. Propranolol,

butalbital. Sumatriptan
succinate, first shot

of what works, rush
of heat through a vein:

surface or depth,
I don't care. Every finger

tingles, bruise blooms
on my thigh. Buys me

days and days. Calculate,
dizzy on the hall floor: more.

6 Galaxies
Grain the trigger, the gut
the gun. Feeding the baby

such a rattletrap trap:
strict dominion

of obscure turns, genes,
lines. Pull the thread

and a stitch
elsewhere twitches, eye

and an eye closing
behind it. Cat's cradle

more skyfield
than map.

We tack spark to spark.
Stars thrum

in the boy's eye. I turn
the cloth again. We wait.

Misalliance

ANITA BROOKNER

Time passed. It was perhaps an hour since she had left the hotel, perhaps an hour and a half. The yellow sky darkened; very occasionally thick drops of rain fell and then stopped. The heated ground drank up the moisture immediately, but from the park came an occasional breath of damp air. In her strange and almost illuminated state of mind, in the airy insubstantiality sometimes conferred by extreme pain, Blanche rested and let her head sink upon her railing. No one seemed to find this extraordinary; there was enough madness about to absorb her aberrant appearance and behaviour. The sight of a woman impeccably dressed yet apparently gazing with fascination at the vibrating side of a Number 36 bus and intermittently bowing her head in prayer caused no ripples of consternation. No one paused in concern or hurried by with averted face; no one hurried at all, but merely passed by in a trance of concentration. Freed by this evidence of the existence of other worlds, of the continued dance of the atoms regardless of her own passivity, Blanche rested her exhausted consciousness. When she could bear to open both eyes she saw merely a darkening sky, and on the other side of the great street a racing stream of traffic anxious to flee the storm.

The taxi, when it came, seemed as exhausted as she herself was; shuddering, it drew up at the railing around which she gracelessly sidled. In the aromatic interior of the cab, its overflowing ashtrays vying with a powerful deodorant, her faintness returned, and her hand crept to her throat as she painfully counted the minutes that separated her from the haven of her home. She was unable, now, to turn her head. Darkness filled the air; it was perhaps nine o'clock. The extreme tension of the atmosphere detonated outbreaks of anxiety in the driver; swerving, he muttered to himself and occasionally punched the wheel with his fist. She was lucky, he told her; he was going home to Putney, turning it in for the night. This was no night to be out. All right, are you? He called back to her. Thought you looked a bit funny. Wouldn't have stopped otherwise. Get you home soon, he said, leaning on the horn. With an enormous effort Blanche opened her mouth. How kind, she said. Tears coursed from her right eye.

In her quiet street, now quite dark, windows shone a golden yellow. Very slowly, her hand supporting her head, Blanche got out of the cab, proffered notes in a nerveless hand, and turned to negotiate the steps of her building. Heavy drops once more fell, hissing on the pavement; a gritty wind had sprung up. 'Mrs. Vernon?' said a voice. 'Mrs. Vernon? Are you all right?' Turning, with infinite caution, Blanche saw Mrs. Duff with some kind of whitish signal in her hand. 'Are you all right? My husband left his newspaper in the car and I came out to get it. I wouldn't have bothered you but you seemed a little strange. Is anything wrong?' Mrs. Duff peered anxiously into Blanche's face. 'Migraine,' whispered Blanche. A hand came out. 'Lean on me, dear. Let me find your key. Never mind, dear. Never mind. You're home now.'

Blanche surrendered to the eternal commiseration of Mrs. Duff, whose sure hand guided her into the stifling stillness of her bedroom, guided her to the bed, and then opened a window on to the rising wind and the random scatterings of the rain. She felt her shoes being removed and a cool damp cloth applied to her forehead. Then there was an absence, during which she knew nothing, a little faintness, a little sleep, perhaps. She was next aware of a whispered conversation: Mrs. Duff had returned with her husband, the dentist, from whose side she never strayed for long. A dark silk handkerchief—the dentist's contribution—was placed over the bedside lamp, and somewhere a kettle was being filled. Then, in the greenish glow of her shaded lamp, she saw Mrs. Duff's face, calm and beautiful with concern. A thin fresh herbal smell filled her nostrils, and a cup was lifted to her lips. 'Drink this,' said Mrs. Duff. Then, sometime later, she said, 'You'll sleep now.' And then, 'I'll look in in the morning. I'll take your key.' 'Come, Philly,' she heard the husband say. 'She'll sleep now.'

But she did not sleep. She drifted in and out of consciousness as if she were moving slowly down a dark passage. Past here glided the kouroi with their blind fixed smile. At some point she managed to get up, to undress, and to put on her nightgown. Then she sank back on to the pillows with her hands tightly clasped, as if in prayer. Sometimes she thought she saw lightning, but could not be sure if it were outside the window or in her head. She was aware of the darkness of the garden, its heavy leafage stirred by the wind, tiny rustlings, the bell round the neck of the stalking cat. At some point she found that she could open and close both her eyes. She lay in a trance of gratitude for her recovered sight, and the kouroi dissolved, taking with them their eternal smile. Once again she got up and felt her way to the window; her face met coolness, night sounds, the order of the universe restored. Sleep remained far off but she did not mind. This night had been given her; she cherished and praised every moment. Some time at around dawn, when the sky began to pale to a whitish grey, she relinquished her hold on her consciousness. At about five o'clock she slept.

When she awoke, it was to an instant of brilliant well-being. Then the dull throbbing started, and she knew that she was in the second phase of her headache. But this was now manageable; she had reached safety. She would simply have to last out the day until the second night, when, she knew from experience, she would sleep heavily. Already she mildly regretted her sleepless night, although she was still stirred by the strange insights that had preceded it. She resigned herself to a day in bed, and looked forward, with childlike trust, to Mrs. Duff's morning visit. There were pills to be taken, ordinary satisfying measures with which to outwit the pain. She thought, like someone who has been ill for a very long time, of the moment of her first bath, of a change of nightgown. The awful evening had left her calm, purged of all imagined obligations. She saw in Mrs. Duff's actions the necessary simplicity of all service, and in her own life of the past few weeks a succession of follies, the origin of which she preferred, for the moment, to leave unexamined.

There was the sound of a key in the lock, cautious steps, the kettle being once more filled. Her door opened slowly, to reveal Mrs. Duff, efficient in navy blue, having clothed herself in quasi-medical severity. They smiled at each other. 'I can never thank you . . . ' Blanche began. 'Thank me? Thank me?' bridled Mrs. Duff. 'If I can't be a good neighbor, and', she blushed at this point, 'a friend, I should like to know what I'm worth.' 'A very good friend,' said Blanche. Mrs. Duff beamed with pleasure. 'Could you drink a cup of tea?' she asked. 'And is there anything you should take?' 'My pills are on the dressing-table,' said Blanche. 'And do come in and have a cup with me.'

This invitation broke Mrs. Duff's hitherto heroic silence, but there is always a price to be paid, as Blanche knew well. During the next hour she heard a great deal about Mrs. Duff's husband's likes and dislikes, her plans for a winter holiday in the Canary Islands ('although he does hate to go away; I have to bully him'), her sister in Oxford who had suffered from migraines as a girl but had grown out of them ('and I never knew what a headache was; aren't I lucky?'), her plans to redecorate her bedroom ('of course, I shall do it all myself'), and her life at home with Mother, who had, surprisingly, been a designer of hats and a court milliner. These revelations had the charm of a fairy tale for Blanche, and although her head ached, she gazed with fascination at Mrs. Duff's fine arched brows, her slightly protuberant blue eyes, and her mobile mouth, the corners of which turned down in unconscious melancholy whenever she stopped talking. Of course, Blanche remembered, there was the little baby who had never come along, no matter how devoted a couple Mrs. Duff and her husband were and had always been. This subject was clearly never far from Mrs. Duff's mind. Presently her eyes filled with tears. 'I saw you with that little girl,' she said. 'For one lovely moment I thought all was well again. You know what I mean. You haven't been very happy, have you?' She dabbed her eyes. 'You must forgive me,' she said. 'Some things you never get over, do you?' She sighed. 'But this won't do. You're the one who needs cheering up. Is there anyone you want me to get in touch with?' 'No,' said Blanche, closing her eyes and feeling suddenly tired. 'Everyone is away.'

Persuading Mrs. Duff to leave and go about her normal day's concerns was no easy task but it was somehow and at length accomplished. Promising to look in again that evening, Mrs. Duff pocketed Blanche's key, picked up her smart straw bag, and left. Alone, Blanche lay back thankfully, but again sleep did not come. It seemed, however, as if Mrs. Duff's reminiscences had banished the antique demons from her interior vision, leaving behind a wistfulness, a desire to have the horizon filled with other figures. A desire also came to her for an impeccable conscience. If I had been a wife like Mrs. Duff, she thought, Bertie and I could have lived as one; instead, I sloped off by myself, and through shyness became quaint. I was not a comfortable person to be with, although I may have been an interesting one. Turning her eyes to the window, she saw drifting veils of rain, for the storm had not broken but had merely retired somewhere else. Weeping skies, and the heavy dark foliage of late summer, made the air in the room seem dense, unmoving. Yet the temperature had noticeably dropped; perhaps the season had ended. The darkness that had filled her vision the night before had perhaps been the true darkness of night falling, rather than the fading vision brought about by her headache. '*Je redoute l'hiver parce que c'est la saison du confort*,' thought Blanche, and comforted herself with pictures of Mrs. Duff as a little girl, playing with her mother's hats, being cosseted by the girls in the workroom, entranced by the women who came for fittings. For she has that intense femininity that comes from growing up in a woman's world, thought Blanche: a world of confidences, secrets, remedies shared. And it has kept her innocent. She knows nothing of the suspect side of femininity, its conspiratorial aspects, its politics. I am sure that she has never engaged in the sizing up of another woman's chances that disfigures so much female thinking; and I am quite sure she has never done that nasty thing, pretended to be sorry for her women friends in the presence of a man. I am sure that she has never needed to mention another woman to her husband, slyly, to gauge his reaction, because, quite clearly, she is the only woman for him. Philly, he called her. Little Philly, trying on the grown-ups' hats. He probably inherited the name from her mother, and so an unbroken chain of affection has nourished her all through her life. I should like to have been a little girl myself; it might have given me more winning ways. But there was always Mother, waiting for me to grow up and take charge, reminding me of onerous duties. Do it now!

Well, I did it, she thought tiredly, and this is where I am. And my conscience is still not clear.

The rest of the day passed slowly and silently. The rain settled down to a steady drizzle, and she heard it pattering on the leaves. At about five o'clock she got up, her eyes weak and smarting, one hand automatically shielding her head. Cautiously she bathed and changed, then got back, shivering, into bed. She reckoned that this might take another day; then she would accord herself the luxury of a day's convalescence. She began to look forward to Mrs. Duff's next visit. Giving Mrs. Duff the key had made her feel trustful, like a child who can expect to be cared for. She even looked forward to the dark, to the drawing of the curtains and the lighting of her lamp, still shrouded in Mr. Duff's green silk handkerchief. When the telephone rang, she was quite surprised; she had not expected to hear from anyone. The bubble of illness in which she was enclosed had seemed to preclude conversations with the outside world. Her pain had required her entire concentration. For all practical purposes she was absent.

'Blanche?'

'Barbara! When did you get back?'

'This afternoon. My dear, the weather was so awful that we began to hate every minute of it. And then that terrible storm last night. That started Jack's foot off again, so we thought we'd get back in case it got any worse. Are you all right? Your voice sounded a bit odd.'

'A headache. I'll be all right in a day or two.'

'Oh dear, I am sorry. You haven't had one for some time, have you? Since that business with Bertie.' There was a silence. 'Perhaps you ought to lie down for a bit. Shall I look in tomorrow. Do you need any shopping?'

'Actually, I'm in bed. And I haven't got a spare key. My very kind neighbour took mine. I'll be perfectly all right in a day or two. It's lovely to talk to you, but I won't talk any more just now, if you don't mind. My voice sounds like a gun to me.'

'My dear girl! Thank goodness I came back. I'll ring tomorrow. If there's anything you need . . . '

'Nothing, thank you. So glad you're back. Love to Jack.'

Lights went on in the corridor; Mrs. Duff had returned. She had changed into a striped silk dress; she probably changed every evening, smartening herself up for her husband's return. She came in, beaming, important, with another cup of tea and some strips of dry toast spread with bitter marmalade, and stood by while Blanche made an effort to eat. When the telephone rang again, Mrs. Duff darted to answer it, listened for a moment, and then said, impressively, 'Mrs. Vernon is unwell. Who shall I say called?'

'A Mr. Fox,' she remarked to Blanche. 'He sounded agitated. He would like you to call him back.'

He might like me to, thought Blanche, but I don't think I will. If he is agitated he can ring his analyst. The person I should ring, of course, is Sally. The thought of Sally brought with it an onslaught of exhaustion. When I'm stronger, she promised herself. When I have decided what to say. For although she remembered every word of the interview at the hotel she had not quite got round to summing it all up. There was unfinished business here, and she did not know how to finish it.

Mrs. Duff placed a jug of lemon barley water by her bed. 'My husband swears by it. I make it myself, of course. And I've left a cold chicken in the fridge and a fruit salad. I dare say you'll be quite hungry by tomorrow. Now is there anything else you want this evening?'

For Mrs. Duff, Blanche could see, was anxious to go next door and cook her husband's dinner: older loyalties prevailed. When she had left, the silence was complete. Darkness had fallen early; the miserable day was over. Leaves dripped outside in the garden. The headache had settled down to a heaviness in the eyes and a sensitivity in the skin of the face and the head; she would be unable to brush her hair for another night. Lying in bed was all that she was required to do, but now she felt less comfortable about it. The sadness of childhood recalled, and the greater sadness that had come with her middle age, turned her thoughts to melancholy and the desire for consolation. In this situation, and unwatched, her brisk mannerisms were of no use to her. They had been summoned up for the benefit of others, of course, and fueled by the wrong sort of pride. She knew now that real pride means gusto; real pride involves fearlessness, bravado, confidence, not a facade behind which one cowers, perplexed, like Adam and Eve in their wretched dilemma, eternal children with a problematic parent they were too inexperienced to challenge. She felt exhausted by the sheer continuity of it all. Wrong start, wrong finish. It was, in fact, characters like Sally and like Mousie who had pride, who went into the jungle of human affairs with nothing but their own weapons to defend them, whereas Paul, now that she came to think of it, had exactly the unthinking placatory attitude that doomed him in his quest for strength. Paul, to a certain extent, was Adam. His trouble was that he had got mixed up in the wrong mythology. Sally (whom she must telephone) would go on to other partners: Paul would be stuck with Mrs. Demuth, with Mr. Demuth always at hand to castigate him. It was a situation which could not be resolved.

And I must stop making stories out of these people, creating false analogies, reifying and mythologizing them, she thought. I have let the National Gallery go to my head. It was this sort of thing that drove Bertie mad.

When she felt stronger (and at the thought she immediately felt weaker) she would telephone Sally, and simply report what had happened. There seemed to be little more that she could do. She might leave another contribution or two under the lid of the teapot, but since she suspected that funds came from elsewhere, she would not make a habit of it. Perhaps Sally would have to be sent off to America to join Paul: this was a very expensive possibility, and yet there seemed no way of escaping from the coils of this dilemma except by extreme actions, such as providing two airline tickets. Surely she was not to be involved to this extent? And yet it seemed likely. It even seemed likely that her conscience was not to be appeased by anything less. Perhaps Patrick might have a better idea, although, knowing Patrick, it would be an idea that favoured non-intervention. Possibly, at this very moment, Patrick was proceeding from Sally to his analyst, or vice versa. The little girl, who had never spoken in Blanche's presence, and who was reputed never to speak at all, was the one to be saved. But Blanche once again saw that she had identified too closely with Elinor, and that Elinor might yet learn those lessons that she, Blanche, had never mastered.

Cautiously lifting her head, she addressed herself to the telephone and dialed Patrick's number. He answered at once, as if he had been waiting for the call.

'Patrick?' she said, in a voice which sounded to her three tones higher than normal. 'It's Blanche. I'm afraid I'm not very well. I won't talk long, if you don't mind.' The telephone hummed with excited silence.

'What news?' asked Patrick, after a short interval, as if he had given her quite enough time to recover.

'Well, I don't really know. I saw those people and they're really quite ordinary, quite respectable. But it's a funny set-up. I think they're keeping Paul on for a bit, taking him back to America. The whole thing is really out of my hands. It was never really in my hands, as you know. I shall certainly not pursue it further.'

'I see,' said Patrick heavily.

'I'll telephone Sally, of course, when I feel a bit better. And then I think it's over to you, if you think you can help. But I would somehow advise against it. Oh, let me talk to you tomorrow or the day after, when I'm myself again. I'm afraid I can't say any more just now.'

'I'm in your debt, Blanche,' said Patrick, in the same heavy tone. 'I have come to a few decisions myself. I will talk with you shortly.'
'Goodnight, Patrick,' said Blanche, and thankfully put the telephone down.

Outside the windows a prematurely black night had established itself. After her conversation with Patrick, the silence was so total that Blanche stirred deliberately in the bed to find out if she could hear herself. It was just as well, she thought, that she was not an hysterical woman. When she heard the key in the lock she could have clasped her hands in a prayer of gratitude. Mrs. Duff had come back, like the Good Samaritan that she was, to say goodnight. But when the door opened, it was to reveal Miss Elphinstone, in her navy blue coat, a plastic rain hood tied loosely over her hat, and bringing in with her usual air of ecclesiastical gentility.

'Good evening, Blanche,' said Miss Elphinstone. 'I was visiting at the hospital, so I thought I'd look in on my way home and see how you were getting on. Terrible weather we had, and not much better here, I see. Black as Egypt's night outside.' And she stepped briskly to the window and pulled the curtains. Immediately the room seemed manageable. Blanche sat up in bed and removed the silk handkerchief from the lamp. 'Shall we have a cup of tea?' she suggested. 'It's good to see you.'

'Well, yes, I could do with a cup,' said Miss Elphinstone judiciously, and went to put the kettle on.

'Well, you look as if you could do with a break and no mistake,' she continued as she came back with the tray. 'In bed at nine o'clock. And that nice chicken in the fridge not touched. Not one of our dishes, by the way.'

'I've had a bad headache,' said Blanche. 'I should be all right by tomorrow. You know how these things go. Mrs. Duff brought the chicken. She's been so kind.'

Miss Elphinstone pursed her lips and drank her tea thoughtfully. 'I'll look in tomorrow and give you a hand,' she said. 'No need to get up if you don't feel like it. You'll want to eat something before you go out on manoeuvres again. Just as well I'm back, isn't it?

'This will interest you, Blanche,' she went on, removing something from her leather hold-all and handing it to Blanche. It was a colour photograph, slightly out of focus, of about eight or ten women, those on the edges of the print indicated by little more than an elbow. 'Taken outside the Bird Sanctuary at Bourton-on-the-Water. That's the Women's Fellowship. Of course, if a certain person had stepped back a bit we could all have got in. I'm naming no names,' she said firmly. 'But what an opportunity wasted. After that the camera got mislaid. But that's another story.'

'It's very good of you,' said Blanche sincerely, for Miss Elphinstone was conspicuous in the middle of the group, leather hold-all well in evidence, worldly smile enhanced by the tilt of an important straw hat. 'You make all the others look frumpish.' For there was something heroic as well as elegant about Miss Elphinstone's demeanour: she could have run a mission station in southern India if she had put her mind to it. She belonged to the days of Empire. She could save a person's life simply by appearing, as she had just now, in the doorway.

'I should say it was a success *on the whole,*' said Miss Elphinstone, retrieving the photograph and giving it a critical glance before putting it away. 'But the weather didn't favour us. And the accommodation wasn't all that commodious. I dare say we shall go back to Devizes next year. And what have you been doing with yourself?'

'Nothing much,' said Blanche, sinking back luxuriously into her pillows. 'Nothing to speak of. It will be nice to get back to normal.' She realized that her notions of normality had become seriously eroded. It was time to get herself back on to a serious footing, whatever that might entail. The alternative was to drift, and that was not to be thought of. It seems that there is still more work to be done, she thought. But sleep was now stealing on her; through half-closed lids she saw Miss Elphinstone's hatted shape standing motionless by the door. And then she thought Miss Elphinstone disappeared, but by this time her eyes were quite shut.

The Migraine Mafia

MAIA SEPP

Right now, my headache is in that muted, dangerous stage where it could go either way; get better, or rampage around my skull like a tantruming toddler. This stage, I like to think of as the squeeze; solid, steady, tortuous pressure. My skin is humming with it.

"I'm glad we were finally able to get together," Avery says, her shoulders hunched in the way of short angry people.

I press my hand against my forehead. "Hmm?" I glance up from my glass to meet her gaze.

"Last time you cancelled at the last minute, so we had to reschedule, remember?"

I do remember. I had a major outage at work which was punctuated by a whopper of a migraine. I've always wondered how Avery can stay irritated at such trivial things for ages when Nate forgets slights the minute they happen.

"Remember?" she repeats. She's holding the spatula in her hand a little like it's a weapon.

"Work stuff," I mumble. "I'm sorry."

"One of your headaches again," she corrects. "I really wish you'd try harder to come to family get-togethers."

"It's dinner, Avery," I say. "It's essentially an excuse to eat a ham."

"It's so much more than that."

"Okay, it's a really *good* excuse to eat a ham." I try to smile at her, to lighten the mood in the tiny room.

Avery stops what she's doing, leaving the oven door open, letting the warmth leak into the already overheated kitchen. It's so close and crowded that it's getting hard to breathe. I pick up the designer purse she gave me for Christmas, which I only use when I come to see her—it's bedazzled—and root around for my all-purpose bottle of pills. If I ever actually packed all the bottles from all the different medications I take there'd be no room for anything else in any of my handbags, so every once in a while I top up a portable pillbox, which, because it's made out of a clear plastic, ends up looking colourful and faintly cheerful. I search for a while before finding the two I want. I usually think of my pills in terms of colour. These ones are blues; over-the-counter, only-sometimes-work blues.

"What are those pills?" Avery leans against the wall and pours herself a glass of wine.

"Nothing." Why, I wonder, didn't I just go to the bathroom and take them there? *Idiot.*

"Doesn't look like nothing."

I sigh. "Your perfume is giving me a headache."

"Don't be ridiculous, smells don't cause headaches." Avery refuses to believe even the most basic science about migraines; she once told me the reason I get them is because I sometimes go to bed at night with my hair wet.

I reach back into my bag and pull out my phone, so I can text Nate to see how much longer he's going to take. After that, I wash the pills down with the soda water. The light in the kitchen is getting brighter, and Avery is starting to look small and far away, like I'm seeing her through a pinhole, and the realization turns my stomach into knots. *Shit.* The tunnel vision and nausea are excellent signs a migraine is on the way. I cover my eyes for a minute, kneading my forehead before running my hand slowly down my face. I try to calm my breathing, smother my worry. Stress always makes things worse.

"You should have a glass of wine, you'll feel better."

Booze with a maybe-migraine? Also not awesome, which Avery's well aware of. "No thank you."

My phone buzzes, and I pull it out of my purse. There's a text from Nate, saying, "Picking up your mom now. There soon."

I don't think I can survive any more time alone with Avery, a thought that makes me sad, albeit briefly. When Nate first brought me home to meet his parents—back when they were in Toronto and Avery was still living with them—she and I got along great. We used to do fun stuff together, go out for drinks every once in a while, have lunch. But I missed returning too many phone calls. Too much work, too many headaches. She finally gave up after I couldn't make her thirtieth birthday party. I always have the best intentions when I see Avery, to get along, to try to spark our old friendship back up. The truth is, I miss her. I glance down; I'm holding onto my glass so tightly my fingers hurt. I transfer it to my left hand and flex out the fingers on my right. Then I take a sip of soda, which lingers in my mouth a lot longer than it should. It's getting hard to swallow now, and all I can think is: *Please don't get worse, please don't throw up, fall down, make a scene.*

"I have a friend at work who used to have migraines," Avery says. "He's totally fixed now! I could get the name of his neurologist."

I try not to sigh. "Sure."

"I'll call him for you." Avery starts chopping onions on a board in her brisk, no-nonsense way. The noise of the knife against the wood is too loud, just too much for the small room. Something rotten darts around my stomach and I shiver. And that's when I know I'm going to be sick.

"Excuse me," I say.

Avery exhales loudly as I walk away. We're not allowed to wear our shoes in her house, so I can feel the nap of the carpet against my feet like sandpaper as I go. Every sensation is amplified now; louder, shinier, squishier than it should be. Instead of using the powder room on the main floor, I go upstairs so Avery won't hear me, and I barely get the door shut before I'm heaving, my face in my hands, my insides burning, my arms shaking. After I'm done throwing up I rinse my mouth out and sit on the side of the bathtub. My legs are so weak I can't stand.

There's a moment where it's just me and the bathroom, cocooned against the world in general and Avery specifically. I put my head down on the bathroom counter, an oasis of cool pressed against my head.

PART IV

It's a Lifelong, Full-Time Job

Introduction

The works in this part focus on the weariness and loss of patience that come from years of migraine, feelings shared by migraineurs, as well as their family, friends, employers, coworkers, and sometimes, even their doctors. Some of these characters and personas have, too, learned tolerance and even acceptance of their relationship with the disease. What most people who have lived with or around migraine for years come to realize is that this disease is part of who the person is, part of how she sees herself and how others see her.

Migraine is not something that turns on and off. Most live with some aspect of the disease all day, every day; it's hard work and often feels like a full-time job—keeping up with appointments to see headache specialists/neurologists for consultations, medications, Botox, nerve blocks, and infusions. Then, there are the different combinations of preventative and abortive medications until the right mix breaks the cycle or keeps the migraineur from moving from episodic to chronic migraine. The many side effects that accompany these drugs are often varied and alter quality of life themselves.

The migraineur visits chiropractors, physical therapists, and other doctors more often than many other people, often because of the deleterious effects medications and the many other symptoms of migraine can have on other areas of the body. Other parts of days are spent wearing the Cefaly device, doing yoga or meditation, and applying moist heat or ice to calm trigger points. Most must find coping methods for dealing with the anxiety, mood swings, communication problems, and depression, which often become part of a migraineur's life.

Part of the job is learning what not to do as much as it is what to do to minimize the number of attacks or the severity of them. There's the need to somehow exercise, despite feeling fatigued and unwell, as well as the choices to make (large and small every day) regarding work, social functions, housework and outdoor tasks, all based on the severity of pain, the potential for pain, and the threat of pain.

Sometimes the work is laborious and tiresome—like walking on eggshells, avoiding every trigger, making choices or decisions based on the weather patterns, making plans for later in the week or month, knowing fully well that the current "good" day has little to do with how she could feel later in the week or even later in the day.

An additional aspect of migraine and its treatment is time: time lost to family, friends, events, and travel. It's also time spent: hours, days, weeks, and sometimes months spent less than whole, lonely and "not normal," clumsy, foggy, looking for words that should be right there. Too much time spent with appointments or on the phone, fighting with insurance companies to allow you to try new treatments, not to cut off care that's desperately needed.

Sometimes family, too, has the sense that if only the setting could change, the familiar routine be left behind, that the migraine and its effects might "go away," perhaps for good. These family members are disappointed when a change of set-ting doesn't make things better. The sufferer can't expect to leave the migraine beyond national and international borders—it comes along. The migraine is the migraineur's fellow traveler. For example, in Andrew Levy's important book, *A Brain Wider Than the Sky,* he acknowledges, "the migraine is my companion now, and I simply can't live without it. It has become my geography, my compass."[1]

Gail Mazur's poem, "Dear Migraine," presents us with a persona who once had similar hopes for mastering migraine by finding new climate and setting, but one who has now learned over so many years, places, and attempts to outsmart the disease, that it's part of who she is and how she lives:

Many times, I've traveled to a dry climate

that wouldn't pander to you, as if the great map
of America's deserts held the key to a pain-free future,

but you were an encroaching line in the sand,
then you were the sand. We've spent the best years

Of my life intertwined[2]

Hilary Mantel in *Giving up the Ghost* remembers a space of seven years, but not in terms of ordinary sentimental reminiscence. For her, the seven years are marked not by normal life events but by the episodes and chapters of her migraine, which include not only the writing she did and the meals consumed but also the thousands of painkillers needed to keep her going during the seven-year period. She is grateful for Mr. Ewing, the one person who understands her, even while she suffers with word blanks, putting sentences and thoughts together. Meanwhile, though, she is all too aware, as are most with this disease, of the difficulty that her disease and all of its manifestations have caused others in her life:

Today, the day I see the ghost, the problem's just that my words don't come out right. So I have to be careful, at Mr. Ewing's, but he understands me without any trouble, and yes, he remembers selling us the cottage, seven years ago, is it really so long? They were years in which perhaps half a million words were drafted and redrafted, seven and a half thousand meals were consumed, ten thousand painkillers (at a conservative estimate) were downed by me, and God knows how many by the people I'd given a pain.[3]

Migraine is associated with substantial disability, low health-related quality of life, and high economic burden. Persons with chronic migraine are also more likely to experience severe disability such as an inability to work, attend social functions, and even perform routine chores.[4] Therefore, this "full-time job" for many precludes any other regular work, which, in turn, naturally leads to significant impact on family, relationships, employers, and coworkers.

This often-disabling disorder accompanies life in the sense that it or the threat of its return is always present. There is a need to increase the knowledge among healthcare professionals about what it means to *live* with migraine.

A study that focused on women's experiences of living with migraine found that the loss of the ability to effectively and clearly communicate is very common:

Not being able to organize thoughts or using the wrong words, as well as not being able to pronounce words because the tongue became numb, [is] embarrassing and add[s]to the feeling of being vulnerable: "It [migraine] affects the whole head. It affects memory. If I'm sitting and talking to people, like when I have guests, and I feel that I'm starting to get a migraine, I think 'What did they say now?' I do not remember. It is like I cannot take it in . . ." This study demonstrates that, "migraine permanently accompanied the women through life, whether by means of its presence or in the form of a perpetual threat that needs to be taken into account."[5]

A major section in Catherine Bush's novel *Claire's Head* is devoted to Rachel's (a chronic migraineur) migraine diary. The beauty of this excerpt is that the reader is able to learn so much about the character's condition, about her nearly lifelong struggle, several times nearly coming to the edge:

A kind of prescience, because of the way you are forced to think ahead. You are always aware this may trigger that—of course I give up trying to think ahead when the endless attention to chains of events proves too exhausting.

And sometimes you push things to the edge, what you do, what you eat, see how far you can go and what you can get away with.[6]

These writers and others in the chapter captivate those of us who already know too well the gripping reality of the disease, but they also serve to enlighten others as to the physical and psychological labor that living with migraine requires; it's like holding down an additional full-time job—one without guaranteed vacations and sick days.

NOTES

1. Andrew Levy, *A Brain Wider Than the Sky* (New York: Simon and Schuster, 2009), 191.
2. Gail Mazur, "Dear Migraine," in *Figures in a Landscape* (Chicago: Univ. of Chicago Press, 2011) 33.
3. Hilary Mantel, *Giving up the Ghost* (New York: Picador, 2003), 194.
4. Amaal Starling and David Dodick, "Best Practices for Patients with Chronic Migraine: Burden, Diagnosis and Management in Primary Care," *Mayo Clinic Proceedings* 90, no. 3 (Mar. 2015): 408–14.
5. Stina Rutberg and Kerstin Öhrling, "Migraine—More Than a Headache: Women's Experiences of Living with Migraine," *Disability and Rehabilitation* 34, no. 4 (2012): 329–36.
6. Catherine Bush, *Claire's Head* (Toronto: McClelland & Stewart, 2004), 213.

An Anatomy of Migraine

AMY CLAMPITT

1

Inquire what consciousness is made of
with Galen, with Leonardo, Leeuwenhoek
or Dr. Tulp, and you find two hemispheres,
    a walnut in a bath of humors,

a skullcapped wreath of arteries, a weft
of fibrous thoroughfares along the walls
of Plato's cave, the cave walls of Lascaux:
    those shambling herds, this hollow

populous with fissures, declivities,
arboreal thicketings, with pairings
and degrees, this fist-sized flutter,
    mirror-lake of matter,

seat of dolor and jubilee, the law of Moses
and the giggling underneath the bedclothes,
of Bedlam and the Coronation Anthem—all
    these shut up in a nutshell.

Go back, step past the nadir of whatever
happened to divide our reckoning, a fraction
of an anti-millennium, a millennium and more
    ago, and hear Hippocrates declare

the brain is double. Since then, as to
where, in these paired hemispheres, the self—
with its precarious sense of *I am I,*
    with its extremes of possibility—

resides, we've come no nearer than
Descartes, who thought he'd found it in
the pineal teardrop. (Now no one's sure
    what that gland is for.)

Inquire what consciousness is made
of Simone Weil, and she answers: Pain.
The drag of gravity. The sledge of time.
    A wretchedness no system

can redeem, extreme affliction that
destroys the *I*; nothing is worse, she
wrote. And knew whereof she wrote, who'd
    drudged, with an ineptitude

only the saints would find becoming,
in a Renault assembly line; had seen
the waste, how small the profit, how
    many suffer and learn nothing, how,

as Kate Croy observed (and chose accordingly),
deprivation made people selfish, left them
robbed of the last rags of character,
    preyed and put upon, enmired in rancor.

She'd seen, was not immune, had been there;
had her own cliffs of fall within the skull:
headache, driven by whose cringing thud
    she'd scrupulously noted

a craven urge within herself to cause
someone, anyone, to suffer likewise.
Is the mind divided, as Hippocrates
    declared the brain is?

Did she invite in what all but unhinged her?
She'd known well-being, however threaded
with crevasses; been witness to the white
    stars' stillness overhead, the white

drift of petals from the apple trees: such
tranquil spanglings of the retina of time,
she could not doubt the universe
   is full, that splendors

of entity, of grace past meeting face
to face, project, each one, its fearful
opposite, its double—as each electron
   in the universe its Manichaean

anti-particle: in every molecule of
every nerve cell, such forces within
forces within forces, the marvel
   is that anyone is ever well,

that consciousness is ever other than
a frazzled buzz, one long sick headache.
My father never gave the name of migraine
   to that locked-in retribution

of the self against—against who knows
what or whom? Fenced brutes, barbed wire
and rawhide, fear of a father's anger,
   mere heredity? His father,

to a grandchild seemingly so mild, so
equable, had labored, I would one day
learn, through that same territory:
   days of headache, nights so worry-

racked he thought his mind would go.
Heredity: finally, in a little memoir
impelled by painful rectitude, he'd
   set down how dread

of what had made him made *his* father
by temper hard: got out of wedlock,
the old conundrum—*Who am I? where did
   I come from?*—twice riddled,

learning whose bastard he was, he'd
manfully assumed that surname. Stirred
or unstirred, the generations' cesspool
    fills; the circle of the wrathful,

ventilated, usurps the crawl space:
all Hell's hand-me-downs hung from
the spindle of Necessity, each sprung-
    from-two, spun-out-of-nothing

being crying from within, *I, I,*
while time that bears the thinking
being toward what it cannot bear
    impales it here.

II

Here is impaled—hinge, mirror-image,
cleft, and crossing-place—the hard
world-knot of entity, the One not one
    at all but contradiction,

Nohow and Contrariwise, chiasmus through
the looking-glass: fraternal inter-
twinings, at the very core a battle;
    so the neurobiological

dilemma of the paired, the hemispheric,
re-ramifies—bright, dark; left, right;
right, wrong—and so euphoria gives way to
    spleen, its obverse, as though

the cosmos repented of itself, of all those
promises, all those placebos: the sun-flooded
square, stone blossoming, each canvas seen as
    a live aperture, a space

to step into; then the usual consequence,
of waking to another migraine: three days
in a darkened room, the drastic easement of ergot,
    derivative of poisoned

rye long known to midwives, proscribed for
her too fragile bloodways. (Lift the hem
of medicine, and you discover torture
    and placebo twinned, still there.)

No cure. This happened, was set down.
I read the manuscript amazed. We hadn't met.
Letters had been exchanged, her driven,
    bannered penmanship an

army out of *Alexander Nevsky*—the whips,
the wolves, the keening steppes, the Russian
mother-lap her history had been torn from.
    One day a parcel came,

impeccably hand-wrapped, inside it an
uncrafted something—three sea-winnowed
sandstones, a wave-buffed driftwood elbow—
    from the beach at Malibu.

I blushed, both flattered and adroitly
remonstrated with: the manuscript (so many
women writing books, their scripts unread,
    still hoping for some recognition!) I'd

said I'd look at not yet opened. I opened
it that day—though not before an ounce
of Maine-coast beach glass had been
    wrapped and sent, transcon-

tinental reciprocity—and read it through.
The migraine on the day she was to fly
to Italy, a frame and a foreshadow
    of that volatile chiaroscuro,

a life repeatedly, strenuously, just barely
put back in order—that migraine (*You too!*)
set her instantly, for me, with an elite
    vised by the same splenic coronet:

Dorothy Wordsworth, George Eliot, Margaret
Fuller, Marx, Freud, Tolstoy, Chopin, Lewis
Carroll, Simone Weil, Virginia Woolf:
   a gathering of shades, of

forebears and best friends who'd all gone
to that hard school. Since Homer peered
at Tartarus, we've looked into a gazetteer-
   authenticated Hell, a place for

meeting with—for hearing yet again the
voices of—the dead. The cosmos, looped with
bigfoot odysseys set down in moon dust, now
   gives it no place but in the hollow

of the skull: that Amazon where no explorer
goes except on hands and knees, the strait
last entrance to the fields of asphodel
   where, say, Simone Weil

and Virginia Woolf might meet and find no distance,
after all, in what they'd finally perceived—
what the latter wrote of as " 'reality' . . . beside
   which nothing matters"; she who'd,

at moments, bridged the mind's crevasse: "Lying
in bed, mad, & seeing the sunlight quivering, like
gold water, on the wall. I've heard the voices of the
   dead here, and felt, through it all, exquisitely

happy." Anny, friend by mail, what I would give
for time to talk of this! We met just once; at ease
at once, walked barefoot on the sands at Malibu,
   the blue air that afternoon, by

some semantic miracle, angelic; picked up stones,
observed the dolphins. A last letter, in that script
her unemphatic beauty stanched without a trace.
   Then, in a hand I did not recognize—

cramped, small, precise—one from the husband
who'd survived her: dead in her sleep. No
warning. But she'd known, had written of, in
    one half-retracted note, a premonition.

I miss her. Though our two lives just touched,
the torn fabric of some not-yet-imagined
prospect hangs there, streamered, splendid,
    vague: well-being rainbowed

over a lagoon of dark: all that I'm even
halfway sure of marked by that interior cleft
(black, white; sweet, sour; adazzle, dim), I
    live with shades of possibility,

with strangers, friends I never spoke to, with
the voices of the dead, the sunlight like gold
water on the wall—electron-charged, precarious—
    all tenuously made of consciousness.

A Brain Wider Than the Sky

ANDREW LEVY

The migraine is my companion now, and I simply can't live without it. It has become my geography, my compass. It comes to Ireland with me when we visit Siobhán's family: the nuanced but never-ending gradations of weather characteristic of the Ulster countryside, for instance, produce nuanced but persistent headaches, most located in the left temple, some over the left eye, oppressive, clumsy, but short in duration, cruising across the noggin from brow to temple like airport runway lights in cascade. . . .

Dear Migraine

GAIL MAZUR

You're the shadow shadow lurking in me
and the lunatic light waiting in that shadow.

Ghostwriter of my half-life, intention's ambush
I can't prepare for, ruthless whammy

you have me ogling a blinding sun,
my right eye naked even with both lids closed—

glowering sun, unerring navigator
around this darkened room, you're my laser probe,

I'm your unwilling wavelength,
I can never transcend your modus operandi,

I've given up trying to outsmart you,
and the new thinking says I didn't invent you—

whatever you were to me I've outgrown,
I don't need you, but you're tenacity embodied,

tightening my skull, my temple, like plastic wrap.
Many times, I've traveled to a dry climate

that wouldn't pander to you, as if the great map
of America's deserts held the key to a pain-free future,

but you were an encroaching line in the sand,
then you were the sand. We've spent the best years

of my life intertwined: wherever I land
you entrap me in the unraveled faces

of panhandlers, their features my features—
you, little death I won't stop for, little death

luring me across your footbridge to the other side,
oblivion's anodyne. Soon—I can't know where or when—

we'll dance ache to ache again on my life's fragments,
one part abandoned, the other abundance—

Giving up the Ghost

HILARY MANTEL

It may be, of course, that the flicker against the banister was nothing more than the warning of a migraine attack. It's at the left-hand side of my body that visions manifest; it's my left eye that is peeled. I don't know whether, at such vulnerable times, I see more than is there; or if things are there that normally I don't see.

Over the years the premonitionary symptoms of migraine headaches have become more than the dangerous puzzle that they were earlier in my life, and more than a warning to take the drugs that might ward off a full-blown attack. They have become a psychic adornment or flourish, an art form, a secret talent I have never managed to make money from. Sometimes they take the form of the visual disturbances that are common to many sufferers. Small objects will vanish from my field of vision, and there will be floating lacunae in the world, each shaped rather like a doughnut with a dazzle of light where the hole should be. Sometimes there are flashes of gold against the wall: darting chevrons, like the wings of small quick angels. Scant sleep and lack of food increase the chances of these sightings; starving saints in Lent, hypoglycemic and jittery, saw visions to meet their expectations.

Sometimes the aura takes more trying forms. I will go deaf. The words I try to write end up as other words. I will suffer strange dreams, from which I wake with hallucinations of taste. Once, thirty years ago, I dreamed that I was eating bees, and ever since I have lived with their milk-chocolate sweetness and their texture, which is like lightly cooked calves' liver. It may be that a tune will lodge in my head like a tic and bring the words tripping in with it, so I am forced to live my life by its accompaniment. It's a familiar complaint, to have a tune you can't get out of your head. But for most people, the tunes aren't the prelude to a day of hearty vomiting. Besides, people say they pick them up from the radio, but mine are songs people don't really sing these days. Bill Bailey, won't you please come home? Some talk of Alexander, and some of Hercules. My aged father did me deny. And the name he gave me was the croppy boy.

Today, the day I see the ghost, the problem's just that my words don't come out right. So I have to be careful, at Mr. Ewing's, but he understands me without any trouble, and yes, he remembers selling us the cottage, seven years ago, is it really so long? They were years in which perhaps half a million words were drafted and redrafted, seven and a half thousand meals were consumed, ten thousand painkillers (at a conservative estimate) were downed by me, and God knows how many by the people I'd given a pain; years in which I got fatter and fatter (wider still and wider, shall my bounds be set): and during seven years of nights, dreams were dreamed, then erased or reformatted: they were years during which, on the eve of the publication of my seventh novel, my stepfather died. All my memories of him are bound up with houses, dreams of houses, real or dream houses with empty rooms waiting for occupation: with other people's stories, and other people's claims: with fright and my adult denial that I was frightened. But affection takes strange forms, after all. I can hardly bear to sell the cottage and leave him behind on the stairs.

Late in the afternoon, a migrainous sleep steals up on me. It plants on my forehead a clammy ogre's kiss. "Don't worry," I say, as the ogre sucks me into sleep. "If the phone wakes, it will ring us." I knew the migraine was coming yesterday, when I stood in a Norfolk fishmonger choosing a meal for the cats. "No," I said, "cod's too expensive just now to feed to fish. Even fish like ours."

The Migraine Mafia

MAIA SEPP

The hold music for Dr. Throckmorton's office is appalling—an instrumental mash-up of a Pearl Jam song that was hip when I was younger but has since been awkwardly transitioned into the world of elevator music. When the receptionist, Shirl, finally picks up the phone she says, "Doctor is busy all day." Shirl sounds even more scrunched than the last time I saw her.

"No problem," I say, rearranging myself a little on the couch. "Can I get an appointment for later this week?"

She makes a noise that could only be described as a snort. A delicate snort, but still. "We're booked for the next three months. I can give you something in January." After the silence stretches she clarifies, "Of next year."

"Okay," I say, pressing my hand against my chest. "I have a problem. I think I might have had a seizure on the weekend, and I'm not sure what to do about this medication she's got me on. Can I just stop taking it?"

"Hold, please."

I look down at my knees, both of them covered with bruises I can't remember getting. I put my thumb on the purple Rorschach of my left knee and watch the colour change. If I was going to take stock of the rest of me I'd be forced to admit I ache with the echoes of my weekend tumble to the tile, the sore elbow, the gimpy ankle, the dent in my pride.

"Hallo?" The voice on the other end of the line is forcefully Eastern European, sort of Bond-villain lite.

"Hello?"

"Yes, hallo, vat I can do for you?"

"I'm not sure," I say. "Because I don't know who you are."

A heavy sigh. "I am nurse practitioner."

"I think maybe you've picked up the wrong line?" I say.

More elevator music rumbles through the phone, a tortured disco tune this time, and I guzzle a glass of water while I wait. My thirst is still sharply intense, worse than I've ever experienced before, and I've had my share of saunas, hot days, and overly enthusiastic sporting events. It's starting to worry me. New prescriptions always make me feel like I'm going through puberty again, and I'm already sick of the constant lab-rat questions I have to ask myself when I'm medicated: is this thirst, dizziness, fatigue, flop sweat normal or is it the new meds? Am I just parched or is the need for water really a sign of something more ominous? I'd much rather focus on things like, how much chocolate am I going to be able to eat today?

To distract myself, I examine the bruise on my other leg. From the right angle it looks a little like Australia. I've always wanted to go—

"Hello?"

"This is Viive Mc—"

"Why are you back at reception?"

"Someone else picked up the—"

"Hold please."

"Hello?" another voice says after a few minutes, a whole new woman.

"I'm Viive McBroom," I say, trying not to sound irritated. "I'm taking an anti-convulsant medication and I think I might have had a seizure this weekend—"

"I doubt that," the voice says drily. "What are you on?"

"Zunosoe, 100 milligrams a day. It's listed as a side effect."

There's a pause, then the sound of keys clicking on a keyboard. "It's highly unlikely. You've only been taking it for a week."

"Right, but it *is* listed as a side effect, and if you Google—"

"Please don't Google," the voice says. "Please don't try to practice medicine. That's our job."

A beat passes, during which I tell myself, *Don't make trouble.* "Anyway, I passed out this weekend, on the kitchen floor. Maybe I fainted, maybe it was a seizure, but—"

"For how long?"

"A few hours."

"Well, it's probably not a seizure." More keyboard clacking. "I have your file here. Just in case, I mean . . . if you really want, I'll call in a prescription for a different type of preventative."

"Still an anticonvulsant or something different? Because I feel—"

"Something in the same family, but with less side effects. What's the number for your pharmacy?"

"One sec."

"I'll put you on hold." Instead, she wraps her hand over the phone and starts chatting to someone. I can't hear them all that well, but it sounds like they're discussing where to have lunch. A loud string of muffled conversation is punctuated by someone yelling, "Purple monkey underpants," and then laughter. "Pharmacy number," the voice says, a few moments later.

"You know, I'd feel a lot better if I could come in—"

"Doctor is booked for the next few months. I'm her intern, I've reviewed your file, and this is standard procedure. Do you have your pharmacy number?"

"Yes," I say, before rattling off the digits.

"I'll call this in now. Have a nice day."

"Should I—"

"Everything will be fine, Mrs. McBroom," she says, just exactly as if she's speaking to a child. "It often takes several iterations before we find a medication that works. And we can't help you if you don't follow our protocol. I mean, how could we?" And then this nameless, faceless person on the other side of the line sighs exasperation into the phone. "Or is it that you don't *want* to follow our protocol?"

I hear the subtext in her voice, and she for goddamn sure knows it. She's mean, this one. I exhale, my heart a quiet thump in my chest. We're now moving into "non-compliant patient" territory, and once they make that assessment they'll never take anything I say seriously, will never really try to help me. I remember that brief moment when I met Dr. Throckmorton, when she seemed confident and knew what I should do. But she's surrounded herself by scrunched receptionists and angry, nameless interns and I can't help but let it shake whatever confidence I might have had in her. *Shit.* Frustration floods through me, the back of my neck surging with heat, tears in my eyes. The silence between me and the intern is suddenly an ugly thing, something actually menacing.

"No, of course not. But I also—"

"Good," she says crisply. "Good day, Mrs. McBroom."

Written the First Morning of the Author's Bathing at Teignmouth, for the Head-Ache

JANE CAVE WINSCOM

WHILST on the beach I stood, my courage fainted,
And busy thought a thousand horrors painted!
Stranger to each, and each to me was strange,
With none a kind 'Good-morrow' could exchange;
With pensive mind, whilst tears my cheeks bedewed,
Fierce Boreas, and a nymph immerged I viewed;
Langour and pain her timid looks express,
As by the women carried in to dress.
'Ah, me!', I cried, 'to plunge into the main
Should I presume, this weak afflicted brain
Will grow deranged, and I shall die with pain!'
But some kind fair, impressed with sympathy,
Consoled my grief, and bade my sorrows flee;
Of whom, to practise what themselves had taught,
One plunged into the sea, with courage fraught;
Near thrice twice-told she dipped quite undismayed,
And then ascends to dress, nor asks for aid.
I chid my fears—my cowardice was nipped,
And next below the wave my head was dipped:
A strange sensation—in a second o'er,
And I quite braced, much happier than before;
When I bathe next, I'll have two dippings more.

O Neptune! should thy waves propitious prove,
And once this grievous malady remove,
Which long has baffled each physician's art,
Moved by the impulse of a grateful heart,
I'll chant thy virtues—sue the tuneful Nine,
And mighty Jove, to lend his aid divine
To fill me with devout poetic fire,
While I to Neptune tune the grateful lyre!

Rachel's House of Pain *from* Claire's Head

CATHERINE BUSH

AUG 15
Keep a record of them, Dr. D. says. A diary. Look for patterns. Any pattern. Keep track of everything you eat, any unusual environments, stresses. I feel like the frog in the pot of water beginning to boil who doesn't know what awaits it but unlike the frog, I'm aware that things didn't use to be like this. I can look back ten or eleven years and although I suffered terrible migraines then, I also know I went out to clubs. I hung out, danced. People smoked. I smoked. I spent hours in bars and didn't think about it. I couldn't have been in constant pain. I couldn't do this now. I remember one night sitting on a bench near the edge of Tompkins Square with Lorrie G., both of us in our little black leather jackets, sharing a flask of brandy (M. must have been away or didn't want to come out) and getting happily drunk. If there was a headache, it came later, and if anything came that night, it must have been something I could toss some codeine at and go on.

AUG 16
2.2 BPS. Right side. Z + Tyl 3(3 a.m.)
I took a lot pills, it's true. More than now? Possibly. I used pills to help me forget the pain, shut it off, so I could go on functioning normally, as if everything were fine. The illusion was that they dissolved the pain but probably they just covered it up. Drugs repress a pain that doesn't want to be repressed.
2.1 Right side. Z + Tyl 3(10 a.m.)

AUG 18
How were things when I was with M.? Before we lived together, I hid things pretty well. Often in the morning, when I got up there would be something so I would down a couple of codeine (222s smuggled from Canada) and eat some breakfast and have a cup of coffee and sometimes the coffee and codeine would act together and I would be fine and sometimes I wouldn't. M. had lost his father when he was fourteen. A heart attack. I wonder if I needed to feel he had access to some sort of pain to feel attraction (I wonder this now, don't think I wondered then). I remember

wanting to seem fearless. I did not want to be the kind of woman who uses pain as an excuse for not doing things. M. used to make fun of what he called an organ recital: old ladies (anyone) sitting around rehearsing their health problems. So, on the whole, I shut up and kept things to myself. And yet he was not unsympathetic. I think he felt his own presence ought to be curative and it was a peculiar kind of insult (he would never have said or even thought this explicitly) when it wasn't.

The first time we met, I felt nothing much. The second time, my heart dropped to my knees. We were at that gallery opening arguing about minimal consciousness, can a rock be said to experience any form of consciousness, if not a rock then a plant, if not a plant then what. His brother was a philosophy professor who studied this. What are the conditions of minimal consciousness? I argued for plants, that minimal consciousness must include some awareness of pain, and the awareness of pain requires consciousness and plants (unlike a rock) are, in some rudimentary way, aware of pain. He started defending rocks. Something about his laugh reminded me of Dad (Of course D was still alive then)—this shook me. If I had a headache that night, I was able to act as if I didn't. He sang. He was taking singing lessons. What son of an Irishman needs singing lessons, he said. He sang Leonard Cohen's "Hallelujah." Because I was Canadian. I have never felt so overtaken by longing as when he walked from one room of my apartment into the other singing in the dark.

If I think back to the headaches then, I was aware there had to be triggers but I didn't know what they were. Sometimes it seemed to be one thing, sometimes another. So I ended up careening about. Anything that seemed to help once—a glass of orange juice, a bottle of Coke—had an almost mystical power. There's a lot of frustration, the sense that you never know how much time you'll have before it begins again. I read with a kind of fury because I never knew how long I had—that probably induced a tension that made everything worse.

Migraines, says Dr. S., are more overdetermined than dreams.

SEPT 21

Today, nothing. Finally. How long will it last? Last week, four days at 2.75 (Barber Pain Scale). (M, T, W, Th) Drugs? (Z + Tyl 3 × 5)

I was trying to finish a piece, past deadline. On how we appear to do, believe we're doing two things at once but on a neurological level, we can't, we switch between them. Only my own crazy brain kept interfering. I'd medicate every four or five hours, but I couldn't get the migraine to cut out, and I had to keep working because they were holding space for me. So sleepy and nauseated, every relevant thought just out of reach, but I had to keep going. I got to the end. Then their e-mail system shuts down or something goes wrong and no matter how many times I send the piece, F. H. doesn't receive it. I don't have a fax machine. I did but it broke. They could have sent a courier but there was worry that the courier wouldn't complete the delivery before the end of the afternoon, and the fact is, I was late and F. was getting pissed off. So I told her I'd bring it in. It's just a subway, a taxi ride uptown and back. I took some Dramamine. If the cab driver or receptionist stared at me strangely I didn't notice. F. doesn't just stare, she asks me if I'm okay in such a way that it's clear something is not okay. At first I think I've slipped professionally. Also, I figure I am nearly green. I touch my hair and scan my clothes but everything seems buttoned right. I tell her I'm fine, just a little tired. This response does not seem to satisfy her. Before leaving the office, I ask for the key to the women's room and check myself out in the mirror. All afternoon, I'd been rubbing the place where the pain was concentrated. I'd rubbed the skin right off. There was a raw, bloody spot in the middle of my forehead.

NOV 2

Woke in night, 3 a.m. After dinner party. 2.25. Z + Tyl 3. Hate explaining to people I barely know why I won't eat something or don't drink. Most people assume you're on a diet or intuit a note of moral superiority. "Don't you have any vices?" a man asked last night.

And then begins a strange, collective, nearly tribal effort to break you down.

Enemas. No vices I will admit to. Okay, it was a wickedly fine Amarone so I broke down, half an inch, that was all it took, half an inch.

NOV 7

Okay today. After that bad day in September, I bought myself a pair of tinted glasses, rose-coloured, since this particular tint is supposed to reduce visually provoked activity in the brain (from fluorescent lights, etc.). Have been wearing them. B. makes no stupid jokes. I did. Yet there's something soothing about the tint, taxis turn to pumpkin, and in no time you forget there ever existed any other colour field. Some days I leave them on until bedtime. Taking them off is a neurological jolt in its own right. Forgot them in a cab today. Trying to decide whether to replace them. Not sure if they work, if they really help, or if I just like them.

FACT O' THE DAY

Dr. Albert Hofmann was working in his lab in 1943 on the ergot fungus, searching for a more effective treatment for migraine, when he first synthesized LSD. No migraine, no LSD. Dr. Hofmann called LSD his problem child, but migraine's mine.

NOV 8

Tension/tension-type headache; chronic daily (mixed, combinations headache, transformed migraine, transformational migraine, rebound headache); analgesic-induced;

cluster; chronic paroxysmal; hemicranias; hemicranias continua; post-traumatic; sinus headache; allergic; eyestrain h'ache; benign exertional; wind in your face h'ache; sex h'ache; ice-cream h'ache; idiopathic stabbing (formerly ice-pick pains); hangover; substance-abuse h'ache; *Lupus h'ache;* Benign cough, external compression h'ache; life-threatening h'ache; fever h'ache; headache caused by malformation of blood vessels; headache caused by lesions; migraine [migraine without aura; migraine with aura (migraine with typical aura; migraine with prolonged aura; familial hemiplegic migraine; basilar migraine; migraine aura without headache; migraine with acute onset of aura); ophthalmologic migraine; retinal migraine; childhood periodic syndromes that may be precursors or associated with migraine (benign paroxysmal vertigo of childhood; alternating hemiplegia of childhood); complications of migraine (status migrainosus; migrainous infarction); migraine disorder (migraines not fulfilling the above criteria)]. Okay, that's enough. This was supposed to be for comfort i.e., thank God, I don't have all of these.

NOV 10

Bad day yest. Walking up First Avenue when a bus went by. All it took. Exhaust, traffic already heavy, air thick. Impossible not to swallow some of it. Pain came on fast. 2.85 on the BPS. Leaned against a lamppost, threw up. Made it home. Usual drugs. Did not used to be like this. Or else the city's getting worse. It makes travel hard but to stop travelling might be the death of me.

NOV 13

Sometimes I rue the day that I ended up in a six-floor walk-up. I could have moved. Seemed like too much trouble. And it's quiet up here. Things would have been so much easier with Star. Now I think: why didn't I? There were lovers who hated climbing stairs and used this as an excuse for our ending up at their place. This was not always a bad thing. And the migraines, so much slamming of the brain with every step.

What if I'd stayed in Toronto? Couldn't have. Stayed with Michael? He wouldn't have stayed with me. Kept Star with me? It would have been worse.

NOV 14

B. asks me if I ever dream about them, a question I have never considered. I said I didn't think I had. I have dreamed about pain. I have dreamed of knife wounds, being stabbed. The dreams of being shot are more about fear than pain. I have dreamed of losing babies, repeatedly. Pregnancies ending in a purge of blood. I have dreamed I am walking through the world with my eyes half-closed and there is nothing I can do to open them. But I've never dreamed of having a headache. (Of sleeplessness, yes, of lying awake, being unable to sleep, and then waking out of this.) Nor can I think immediately of something that would be an obvious stand-in for such pain. Nor do I know, now that I think about it, if it would be possible to dream about pain directly, although I have been hungry in dreams, and woken myself, out of dreams, to terrible pain. Always the hunger. When the pain is still small, and before the nausea sets in, the hunger begins, it rumbles up, and when I eat, I'm soothed a little, though this, too, is a chemical reaction, and the hunger returns and grows until I feel insatiable, and then the sole of my right foot begins to ache, like a warning, a bell tolling, the sensation travelling all the way up the interior of my leg into my back and into my neck.

Yet the hunger is also a kind of ecstasy. It leads to sex. Claire says she can't have sex when she has a migraine but sometimes what better way to forget, find release, be desired, convince yourself the body is something other than a conduit for pain. There is a difference. I mean, when it gets really bad, there's no point, obviously.

The difference between migraines and sex. At the heart of a headache, when pain overwhelms you, is the desire for stillness, internal and external, whereas sex is about motion, sensation through motion, sensation existing along a spectrum of pleasure and pain. There is no way to confuse migraines and sex.

S., always, a little nut inside me.

NOV 18
I have joined a pain support group. In the spirit of trying everything before giving up, I went for a second time to a meeting of a pain support group. You're supposed to describe your pain(s) and talk about what you've been through recently, the theory being that talking about this among people who have some similar understanding will begin to make it all seem more bearable. The woman who coordinates the group, Nicki Sanchez (assisted by this old arthritic guy named George) drives me crazy. She's very tall and stoops because she obviously thinks herself too tall and half covers her mouth when she speaks. You can practically feel the tension in her muscles, which must at least be part of her problem, so visibly tense I want to shake her. And when she doesn't think you're looking, she's busy pushing her fingers against her body, all over, which of course looks strange, like she's continually poking herself, but I know exactly what she's doing, she's pressing on points that hurt. If nothing else, I tell myself, I'm here for the stories: girl in a car accident, younger than any of us, not obviously hurt, but ever since has suffered terrible ringing in her ears, so loud much other sound is blocked out, which I accept as a form of pain. Met

another migraineur, guy, so photosensitive in the midst of an attack that he can read books (not that he feels like reading) in the dark. No mention of higher powers, thankfully. We are simply here to commune with each other.

I have also realized there are no people here on crutches or with obvious wounds. The flyer on the street said nothing but Pain Support Group. Perhaps we with our invisible pain are the most desperate. We sit in a circle (hideous). Tonight, they asked me to stand up and speak about my experience and because I am new everyone was very gentle and supportive. I couldn't do it. I stood and said, Those who don't feel pain are freaks.

NOV 21

Kim Stuckless called. Haven't spoken to him in at least twelve years, since he moved to New Zealand. He said he's coming to NYC in February and wants to get together. I said as far as I know I'll be here. He's bringing his eleven-year-old son, Max, who gets migraines with auras. Whenever the aura begins, Max says to Kim, the men are coming. He sees men. Until a year ago, his migraines had only ever occurred on the left side. The one thing that relieved them without medication was going to really loud rugby matches. Last year Kim brought Max back to Toronto for the summer. When they changed global hemispheres, Max's migraines switched brain hemispheres, left to right. The whole time he was in Canada, they were consistently on the right side, but when he returned to Auckland, the migraines switched sides once again.

NOV 22

2.30 (yest), R side, came back, this a.m. L side. Bad. Usual drugs.

NOV 24

Hildegard von Bingen, Joan of Arc, Julius Casear, Cervantes, Blaise Pascal, Alexander Pope, Immanuel Kant, Frederic Chopin, Friedrich Nietzsche, Sigmund Freud, Thomas Jefferson, Lewis Carroll, Virginia Woolf, Joan Didion.

NOV 25

It always strikes me how few women are on these lists, even though statistically far more women get migraines than men, so does this mean, historically, that more men got migraines (unlikely), or (more likely) those few women who figured out how to make productive use of their painful selves (subverting diagnoses of hysteria) kept their mouths shut about their pain. Do men in pain achieve more than men who do not suffer recurrent pain? Freud tried cocaine to treat his.

No men in our family get them—only women. Right down the female line: my great-grandmother, grandmother, mother. Who knows when it began. In evolutionary terms, they must have had some protective value. A strategy. Dr. S.'s theory: a response to external threat. My grandmother called them sick headaches. She had them badly but only occasionally. Like my mother. So what happened to make ours so much worse? Not just me, one freak, but me and Claire.

Sometimes I wonder if we're more aware of pain because we're so inundated by external stimulation and change, which wear our resistance down. We are so overloaded we've lost our filtering mechanisms, or is it the reverse, because we have so many fewer physical distractions we have more space for this kind of pain. We feel more because we suffer less, because we no longer expect to suffer continuously, because we live in the expectation of being pain-free. It's a luxury to be able to complain. Either that or we're doing something really wrong. (Notes towards a philosophy of—)

NOV 27
They're not getting better. Maybe I'm imagining they're getting worse. 2.5 this a.m. In our family, there was no obvious advantage to being sick. You did not get more attention. When I was eight, I was fascinated by nineteenth-century women (Helen Keller, Laura Bridgeman) who were blind, deaf, and mute. Their condition seemed so extreme I limped for a while, on purpose. I suppose it was a way of making myself more aware of my body.

When I ran, but then it was more about strain, on the way to achieving something, there was payoff, at least until my knee fucked up.

NOV 29
My father wanted me to become a doctor. And in the beginning I did not entirely rule it out, since I was in sciences but it soon became clear to me that I simply wouldn't be able to do it. The day I told him I didn't think I'd ever be able to hold a full-time job, he yelled at me to stop being such a snob and I yelled back that he had no idea, absolutely none, what it was like. He was the one who was supposed to become a doctor. He was the one for whom sacrifices were made. They came to Canada because they believed it would be easier for him to practice here, get him out of the slums of East End London, where of course it had been impossible for his father to become a doctor, however much he wanted to and apparently he did, but he had to stay in the family shop, he had no choice, the youngest, all his brothers killed off in the first war so really there was no choice. Dad was the first one to go to university. He was the first to have a chance to become a doctor, and in the beginning it seems he genuinely wanted this (not that there's anything socially regressive about becoming a teacher). Was it entirely because of J. B., because of the horror of her death and helplessness in the face of it, that he quit? (But he

didn't quit then, he took a term off from school, went back.) So what happened later—why quit after he'd met Mum, after she became pregnant with me? He got sick and had to take more time off school, but if he left simply because he'd gotten behind, why didn't they say that? No, there must have been some kind of crisis, a loss of faith. Was it discovering himself with another woman with a chronic if less debilitating condition? Was his mind already mostly made up and it took only one more trigger, this small thing, this other helplessness, to push him to the brink?

What gets passed on? My parents die a freakish, grisly death but my grandmother watches her mother die in front of her. She's twenty-one. After her mother has a stroke and collapses at the dentist, she manages to get her home by tram, because there are no taxis or ambulances in their town, but the doctor's taken the afternoon off and her father's at lunch and she can't get her mother upstairs into bed. Somehow she manages to manoeuvre her into an armchair in the living room. Then she dies. They both (M & D) lived through the war. I asked Dad what it was like when the fighter planes flew over his head in Oxted and said after the first rush of terror he felt a kind of excitement. But there was another time, before this, when he was still in London. There was some kind of metal cage set up in the living room for them to sleep in, to protect them if the house was bombed. And he was put to bed in there one night with a blanket or a tablecloth thrown over top. For some reason Al, the baby, was not inside, he was with their mother. It wasn't late. Granddad B., who was a warden, was around. An air-raid siren goes off and they race for the shelter down the street. Grandma B. must have thought Granddad would bring Hugh. Whatever. In the shelter, she discovers Hugh isn't there and flips out. That night something hits very close to them. When they're finally allowed out, they discover the house next to theirs has been demolished and their house is only partly standing, the front wall with the door still in place, the back a mess, the living room covered in debris but the cage still there (covered in dust, etc.) and when they pull off the cover, there is Hugh, sleeping. He was not, apparently, concussed, he was simply asleep. A reaction to shock, presumably. They had to shake him and shout his name to wake him up. That's trauma but I drink milk and it brings on a headache.

DEC 5

We met for dinner. I had no expectations. The plan was to talk about pain and his photosensitivity, which interested me. It's a strange kind of bonding, but one I respond to and at that moment that was all I wanted. Partway through dinner, he took off his jacket. His arms were bare. Chinese script ran up the inside of both arms from his wrists towards his armpits. He told me it had taken two days to get the tattoos done, one arm one day and the other the next, and on the day in between he almost decided not to go back, although the whole point of this pain was that it was consensual. He got them done after he ended up in hospital once—

status migrainosus. Days and days with absolutely no break at all. He was ready to kill himself. They threw narcotics at him, doped him to sleep. He said, it's true, you don't get high. I said I'd ended up in hospital once or twice but not for years and these days I wasn't sure I saw the point, but we had this between us now, the awareness of what it's like to be so close to the edge that there is almost nothing else of the self left. There's something arousing and sensual about recognizing that state when you are not in it (been there and returned), recognizing it in someone else (empathy without pity or indulgence). Then it is possible to feel vulnerable. I wanted, I needed to feel those arms around me. He said (we were in bed by then) that when the pain is terrible, he holds up his arms in the dark (he held up his arms) and reads from them, and I can't repeat the characters or how they sounded, but these were the phrases, he said, that kept him from killing himself.

Have retreated from B., but also from everyone, from everything.

DEC 9

If he called me and said, come to me, it will help, I would go—but no matter how awful I feel, I cannot call him. The world feels so distant, the sky, the water towers on rooftops, the pigeons, the guy playing the trumpet on another rooftop (an oddly warm day), the sound of buses. Bad but a little better now. 2.whatever. Still bad. Things fall away, the deadline for that article, the desperate need to eat in that restaurant on First Street, whether B. will drop by, the gnawing fact that I should call S. It is not only the self that feels fragile but the world, so little holds it together and binds me to it. It would be so easy to disappear. A bad migraine is a little death.

DEC 10

A kind of prescience, because of the way you are forced to think ahead. You are always aware this may trigger that—of course I give up trying to think ahead when the endless attention to chains of events proves too exhausting.

And sometimes you push things to the edge, what you do, what you eat, see how far you can go and what you can get away with, because how is it possible to live without testing, hoping. And then you pay for it.

Sometimes I think if I can describe it, that will help. It is like a fit of depressive mania, or at least a fit of depressive mania is like an inversion of a migraine, a migraine without the pain. First the torpor. Then the loss of appetite (rather than hunger). The disgorging of the body. The catatonia and internal wildness of complete despair. The knowledge that it will pass even as it seems impossible, inexplicable that it will ever pass. Like lost love. You cannot see the way out. You have no idea how you will get out. But the next morning dawns, bright and ordinary again.

DEC 11

2.95 on the BPS. Day three on R side. Muscles hurt. Why so much worse now? They were bad after Star's birth, very bad. There were days when I'd look at her and barely be able to see her. I'd walk towards her and feel like I was walking through a flood, limbs barely part of me. How hard it was to respond to her as a human being when in this state, to do even the ordinary things, lift her, feed her, bathe her.

This offers some comfort. It is chaotic but not random. It begins in instability. It is a complicated, dynamic system of neural behavior and response. You tip from an unsettled state into illness, and at certain critical times, it takes only the smallest stress to push you from unsettledness into illness. Each thought, each action, everything you eat functions as a neuro-chemical threshold, you move through thresholds towards the final threshold, the singularity, something so small, possibly infinitesimal, that pushes you over the edge.

But the problem, neurologically speaking, is complex, for how much of the migraine is other and how much is indissolubly, chemically part of the self. For instance, a mathematician who suffered from severe migraines went to a neurologist after many years of agony and somehow he managed to locate her single trigger—cheese, say cheese—and all at once when she stopped eating cheese, her headaches vanished but just as suddenly she lost her ability to do higher mathematics. Something about her mathematical genius was so chemically or structurally connected to whatever created the migraines in her brain that she had to choose, pain plus mathematics or no pain and no math. She took the pain and chose the math.

If you can't feel pain, you die. This offers some consolation, if not exactly comfort.

Sonya calls. We make plans to meet for dinner. We haven't seen each other for months, which is largely my fault because I haven't been returning calls. So it's a little awkward. When we meet it's clear how happy she is, she can't hide it and once we're sitting down in the most smoke-free place we can find, she tells me she's pregnant. She's embarrassed, I think, because she's not sure how I'm going to respond. She knows what I did, giving up S. I don't know if she can forgive me for it. I don't know if I can forgive myself. We don't speak of it but it's there between us. I tell her I'm glad for her, after so long (she's convinced it's partly due to her work with A.), and I am, of course I'm glad.

Perhaps it helps to think of the worst. To place the worst in the past. The day M. and I arrived in Ethiopia (the trip we'd planned for ages—I wanted to take him to the place I'd come to consciousness, so much more meaningful than the place where you're born). We landed at the same time as the Chinese prime minister's Official Delegation, and so were kept on board for hours more after a ten-hour flight while the airport was emptied for their arrival and they were heralded across the tarmac by a military marching band, glimpses of which we could see through our airplane windows, so that I was not in good shape by the time we finally made it into the terminal building and into an interminably long and slow line, and grew worse while we waited and I was so ill and addled by the time we got to the customs official (already vomiting, occasionally racing to a sour but functional toilet and unable to keep any medications down) that he kept asking us more and more questions, which lit the long fuse of M.'s annoyance, (I wasn't sure the customs guy was going to let me in the country), and by the time we made it out to where Mum's friend Eileen was frantically waiting, as she had been for hours, behind a barrier, outside the terminal, because of the reception of the Official Chinese Delegation, and into her white Pajero, I was repeatedly throwing up into the only plastic bag I'd managed to rustle out of my luggage, completely dehydrated, (soldiers everywhere), M. furious, Eileen looking nervous about the state of me (collapsed on the back seat) and M. and her truck, (none of this like what she'd anticipated) as we drove along behind the marching band—in other words a real doozie that lasted about five days out of our ten-day trip, and I remember thinking then, for the first time, it will end, Michael and me, not now, but it will end.

One year, at the opening party for the Whitney Biennial, I spent most of the evening lying on a small black-cushioned bench in the dark womb of a video exhibit.

Once I had to drive alone into the city in heavy, rush-hour traffic across the George Washington Bridge, drugged, barely able to keep my eyes open, stuck in the outside lane, the river beneath, and I thought, I can't go on like this, it would be so easy to—there was nothing to do but keep driving.

I've survived all this. Such solitude, such humiliation to this kind of pain and, even as you're aware of the humiliation, such detachment.

I remember the hospital visits and I remember so many rooms, so many hotel rooms, by their ceilings. Green hotel ceiling in Shanghai. Light fixtures, ceiling fans. Why travel if it's so hard? Because every time you go somewhere else there's a chance of throwing yourself in the path of something unforeseen. These days I check out the state of bathrooms, of toilets, first thing, given the odds that I may be kneeling in front of them. Sometimes even clean them—me—if they're particularly disgusting and it looks likely I'll be sticking my head in.

Sometimes when I lie in bed, it's as if there's a figure at the other end of the bed whispering, what will you give up to be free of it? And I'm convinced, if only I can find the right thing—I have given up so much. How much more can I give up?

Or I think my only hope is a kind of continual neurochemical track-switching, a shape-shifting, go suddenly off medications, change diet, change anything that will allow me to restart, to outsmart, if only temporarily, the pain grooves.

Someone once said. It is like you have a ghost living inside you.

M. once said, You should get a new head.

Is there some essential part of me that isn't touched by pain, or, no matter how many layers you peel away, is it still there, a thought which depresses me, but also comforts, *because* it makes the pain essential.

B. has a way of asking, Do you have a headache, that is less judgmental than anyone I have known. He manages to make an observation without any trace of blame or recrimination, not the subtlest nudge of what have you done now?
    (And yet I'm frightened of his pity. If this gets worse, it will come.)

I told him about R.H., the man from the pain group. He freaked. Perhaps that's what I wanted. Why are you so cruel, he yelled. I suppose I wanted to hurt him—perhaps it's all I can bear. I want to feel helpless. I want not to.

The thing is, I sleep better when I'm with B. than almost any other time.

JAN 2, 2000
I feel saturated with her ever since I got back. She's learning to draw Chinese characters, Len's teaching them, he's bought them special exercise books. She showed me hers at Xmas. I made a mistake, though, near the end. I asked her if she wanted to come live with me. I asked out of curiosity just to see how she would respond and her face took on the most peculiar expression. She doesn't want to, she was frightened I was going to take her away but she also wanted to placate me because she knows I have the power to take her away and she doesn't want to hurt me because she loves me and so felt she should say yes (she wants to want to) but she couldn't honestly. Maybe, she said. I said, Don't worry, I'm not going to. I said I thought she was happier with her cousins. I wanted to walk through a door and vanish. Ravaged. The wind knocked out of me. Whatever I do I have failed her. If I took her back now I could not change my mind ever again. And how could I look after her now, like this? I made an agreement. She doesn't remember living with me. (Sometimes she seems as far away as a dream, sometimes I miss her so much I cannot see what's in front of me.) She says she remembers the bed. I remember her sleeping beside me, how restless she was, how restless we both were. I remember the smell of her scalp

and her ears. I remember lying on the floor of the front room with a headache, for hours, not wanting the weight of her presence beside me. Working at night in the front room, I'd walk past the bed on my way to the toilet and be shocked at the sight of her. For the first year there was such joy in her presence, my little love, and wonder, and I'd think of calling her father to say, look what we've made (the pure gift—the extraordinary openness of those moments on the train), but I didn't (and now I can't call him, because how can I admit what I've done?). What did I dream would happen? I dreamed things could be different. I dreamed the pain would break because it had to. But it didn't. I began to weep at the thought of hauling her down and up the stairs. I'd imagine the two of us leaping out the window just to see if there was an easier way of getting from here to there. That winter, the pain was making me crazy, it makes you crazy, all I could think was what could I give up, I had to give something up, I would have given up anything if it made the pain go away.

JAN 3
S. calls. Mother, she says, listen to our spell. I am so miserable, make me invisible. But she's laughing, they're all laughing, I can hear them.

JAN 15
Have been boiling up herbs like a witch.

JAN 30
There are two places in the world that may offer the migraineur sensitive to me-terological and barometric fluctuations some sustained relief: the middle of the Dead Sea and the bottom of the Grand Canyon.

FEB 6
Dr. D. suggests Botox. Says he has nothing else left to offer. Ladies who use injections of the botulism bacterium to relieve their wrinkles by freezing their muscles have discovered it helps their migraines. They think it works by numbing the area around the trigeminal nerve. Injections last about three months. It costs c. $500 a pop. I ask about side effects. None, he says. Well, your eyebrows may collapse.

FEB 10
Claire said she thought I might go for it.

I cannot eat any dairy products at all now. I am needless to say assigned to write an article on the wrinkle-free wonders of Botox. I try to avoid walking along streets that are bus routes or which have a lot of truck traffic. I suppose I could try wearing a face mask as the Japanese do when sick. Even in Manhattan the prospect daunts me. I can last about five minutes in a dry cleaner's. I wave from outside the door of the place across the street on 9th and hang what clothes I do dry clean in the bathroom with the window open for a day. I stay clear of people wearing strong perfume, especially in movie theatres. Avoid movie theatres. Newspaper ink's a problem, but depends on the newspaper. *Times* still okay. Sugar. Dairy. Smoke. Alcohol. The smell of onions. Carpets, esp. new ones made of petroleum-based substances. Oil paint. Varathane. Bleach. Air on airplanes. Muscles hurt. Worse on days when head's less. Maybe it's New York. Maybe it's the life I lead. Maybe it's the world and I'm a canary in it. Everything feels toxic. Yet I am a lucky woman. I can still afford my health insurance, and the bloody Zomig, which isn't working as well as it used to but soon there'll be a new generation of drugs. I have money, work, nothing to complain about. It's all in my head. In all likelihood I'm not dying any faster than anybody else.

Woke thinking of M & D. Wake at the first signs of pain, fearing it will grow. It will grow. Take drugs. More drugs. Think of them on the escalator, riding up. Let them have been happy together at the end. (How many times have I flown through Frankfurt and yet never been on that escalator.) I hope she didn't have a migraine. I think of the photos he took of her in High Park, the day he asked her to marry him, the ones he loved and she hated because she had a migraine. Did he know this about her then?

I could pray. Try to believe suffering is worth it for its own sake.

What is the opposite of pain? Some other kind of pain?

Think of it as fluid. Think of it as your medium, said A. Works for a while. In the doorway, he kissed me on the lips, which surprised me, but I don't think it was a sexual kiss.

Arms hurt too, not so bad on days when my head aches. What lurks always are the things that cannot be said.

There's no use keeping a headache diary expecting it to reveal patterns of cause and effect.

Is the key, still, to give something up, then what, what is the thing to give up?

Three, okay, three, three, three, Fuck the Barber Pain Sale.

Arms at Rest

SIRI HUSTVEDT

I am a migraineur. I use the noun with care, because after a lifetime of headaches, I have come to think of migraines as a part of me, not as some force or plague that infects my body. Chronic headaches are my fate, and I have adopted a position of philosophical resignation. I am aware that such a view is resoundingly un-American. Our culture does not encourage anyone to accept adversity. On the contrary, we habitually declare war on the things that afflict us, whether it's drugs, terrorism, or cancer. Our media fetishizes the heart-warming stories of those who, against all odds, never lose hope and fight their way to triumph over poverty, addiction, disease. The person who lies back and says, "This is my lot. So be it," is a quitter, a passive, pessimistic, spineless loser who deserves only our contempt. And yet, the very moment I stopped thinking of my condition as "the enemy," I made a turn and began to get better. I wasn't cured, wasn't forever well, but I was better. Metaphors matter.

Although I wasn't diagnosed with migraine until I was twenty, I can't remember a time when I didn't suffer from headaches. A German neurologist, Klaus Podoll, who has studied migraine auras and artists, contacted me a few years ago after he read an interview I had given, in which I mentioned a hallucination that preceded one of my headaches. In an e-mail conversation, he questioned me carefully about my history and concluded that the annual bouts of what my mother and I thought were stomach flu were probably migraine attacks. I have come to agree with him.

My "flu" was always accompanied by a severe headache and violent vomiting. It didn't occur during the flu season, and the sickness always followed exactly the same course. Two days of pain and nausea that lightened on the third day. Throughout my childhood, the attacks came with ritual regularity. In high school, I didn't have as many "flus," but after I returned from an intensely exciting semester abroad, spent mostly in Thailand, during my third year of college, I fell ill with what I thought was yet another flu, a siege of excruciating head pain and retching that lasted six days. On the seventh day, the pain lifted somewhat, but it didn't go away. It didn't go away for a year. It was better; it was worse, but my head always hurt, and I was always nauseated. I refused to give in to it. Like a dutiful automaton, I studied, wrote, received the desired A's, and suffered alone until I went to my family doctor, sobbed in his arms, and was diagnosed with migraine.

My young adulthood was punctuated by the headaches with their auras and abdominal symptoms, nervous storms that came and went. And then, after I married the man I was deeply in love with when I was 27, I went to Paris on my honeymoon, and fell sick again. It began with a seizure: my left arm suddenly shot up into the air, and I was thrown back against the wall in an art gallery I was visiting. The seizure was momentary. The headache that followed went on and on for month after month. This time I searched for a cure. I was determined to battle my symptoms. I visited neurologist after neurologist, took innumerable drugs: cafergot, inderal, mellaril, tofranil, elavil, and others I've forgotten. Nothing helped. My last neurologist, known as a headache tsar in New York City, hospitalized me and prescribed Thorazine, a powerful anti-psychotic. After eight days of stuporous sedation and an ongoing headache, I checked myself out. Panicked and desperate, I began to think that I would never be well.

As a last resort, the tsar sent incurables like me to a bio-feedback man. Dr. E. hooked me up to a machine via electrodes and taught me how to relax. The technique was simple. The more tense I was the louder and faster the machine beeped. As I relaxed the sounds grew slower until they finally stopped. For eight months, I went for a weekly visit and practiced letting go. Every day I practiced at home without the machine. I learned how to warm my cold hands and feet, to increase my circulation, to dampen the pain. I learned to stop fighting.

Migraine remains a poorly understood illness. Although new techniques, such as neuroimaging have helped isolate some of the neural circuits involved, brain pictures won't provide a solution. The syndrome is too various, too complex, too mixed up with external stimuli and the personality of the sufferer—aspects of migraine that can't be seen on M. R. I. or PET scans with their colored highlights. I have come to understand that my headaches are cyclical and that they play a part in my emotional economy.

As a child, life with my peers in school was always hard for me, and my yearly purges no doubt served a purpose. For two days a year, I suffered a cathartic dissolution, during which I was able to stay home and be close to my mother. But times of great happiness can also send me over the edge—the adventure in Thailand and falling in love and getting married. Both were followed by a collapse into pain, as if joy had strained my body to its breaking point. The migraine then became self-perpetuating. I am convinced that a state of fear, anxiety, and a continual readiness to do combat with the monster headache pushed my central nervous system into a state of continual alarm, which could only be stopped by a deep rest. I continue to cycle. Periods of obsessive and highly productive writing and reading that give me immense pleasure are often followed by a neurological crash—a headache. My swings from high to low resemble the rhythms of manic-depression or bipolar disorder, except that I fall into migraine, not depression, and my manias are less extreme than those of people who suffer from the psychiatric illness.

The truth is that separating neurological from psychiatric problems is often artificial, as is the old and stubborn distinction between psyche and soma. All human states, including anger, fear, sadness, and joy are of the body. They have neurobiological correlates, as researchers in the field would say. What we often think of as purely psychological, how we regard an illness, for example, is important. Our thoughts, attitudes, even our metaphors create physiological changes in us, which in the case of headaches can mean the difference between misery and managing. Research has shown that psychotherapy can create therapeutic brain changes, an increase of activity in the pre-frontal cortex, the "executive" part of our mind organ. Yes, just talking and listening can make you better.

No one ever died of a migraine. It isn't cancer, heart disease, or stroke. With a life threatening disease, one's attitude—whether bellicose or Buddhist—cannot keep you alive. It may simply change how you die. But with my migraines that continue to arrive and no doubt always will, I have found that capitulation is preferable to struggle. When I feel one coming on, I go to bed, and now machineless, I do my relaxation exercises. My meditations aren't magical, but they keep the worst pain and nausea at bay. I do not welcome my headaches, but neither do I see them as alien. They may even serve a necessary regulatory function, by forcing me to lie low, a kind of penance, if you will, for those other days of flying high.

PART V

When It's Gone . . .

Introduction

"When It's Gone . . . ," perhaps more than the other parts, speaks most directly to the migraineur. After all, the family and friends, doctors and students all benefit from the "lifting" of a migraine or the at least temporary resolution of one—but none more so than the migraineur. When the migraine finally subsides, and the worst of the throbbing, seemingly endless headache pain finally recedes, most migraineurs experience a migraine "hangover," a time (sometimes for a day and often longer) when the neck feels like it cannot hold up under the incredible weight of the head, which seems to weigh a ton. The fatigue is unlike any other, and the body feels like lead. There is a level of grayness, a real inability to feel much of anything and certainly still the loss of certain cognitive functions.

For some, though, the migraine actually seemingly "lifts" from the body, and, in those times, one finds an exhilaration, a joy for life not often experienced. There are these exceptional moments, maybe even days or weeks, when the whole of the migraine episode leaves, lifts from the body and the psyche. We rejoice; pain, heaviness, fatigue, and overall illness are replaced by exhilaration, lightness, and an abundance of gratitude. Many writers, including Virginia Woolf and Anna Leahy, speak directly to the full presence and energy with which we then experience every ordinary moment, sight, or even sound. Andrew Levy reminds us that while the pain is indescribable, "joined to that pain, rising from it like a phoenix, it is also a story about hope."[1]

For most chronic migraineurs, though, the thoughts right after first experiencing the joy of a migraine finally lifting are: How long will this relief last? How careful do I need to be? I have so much to do, in case it comes right back. The fear is deep and real, and we struggle not to let it overwhelm the beauty, joy, and lightness that have come from the migraine finally leaving the body. Perhaps what makes this respite so poignant and seemingly indescribable to others is, in part, because we don't know how much time we will have before the next episode begins. Such awareness is a topic Anna Leahy addresses in her essay: "I'm usually not sure when that next migraine will be, but I expect it to come. I have an unknown timeframe between migraines and can't procrastinate."[2] Sometimes, too, we make plans during these good times, always keeping in the back of our minds that there's the distinct possibility that a new episode could well have begun by the time the event arrives. These fears are the ones with us on the good days.

When we experience respites, however long, without migraine, we know there will be another, but it is how we spend the time we are symptom-free that matters, that keeps us going, that gives us hope. Gavin Ewart's poem, "The Night-Rider," echoes the composer Sibelius's tone poem of the same name, in which the night rider travels through darkness and "painful lightnings" until meeting the eventual light:

> If you ride long enough
> you come to sunrise,
> to a gentle, natural light
> that could hurt nobody,
> sunshine and birdsong.[3]

We are "night riders," whether riding to get to the end of one cycle or episode and eventually getting there, or riding to get to that treatment or combinations of treatments that bring us long-term improvement of quality of life.

Significant research and studies now devoted specifically to migraine are providing our headache specialists/neurologists so much more understanding about what actually happens in the brain before and during migraine episodes and in the brains of people with migraine disease. We are living in promising times for new treatments—the first-ever devices and medications created just for people with migraine, including the recently available CGRP inhibitors: "The solution is partly / to keep on riding."[4]

NOTES

1. Andrew Levy, *A Brain Wider Than the Sky* (New York: Simon and Schuster, 2009), 233.
2. Anna Leahy, "Half-Skull Days," *The Pinch* (Spring 2012): 154.
3. Gavin Ewart, "The Night-Rider," in *Night Ride and Sunrise*, ed. Edward Lowbury (Aberystwyth, Wales: Celton Poetry, 1978), lines 18–22.
4. Ewart, "The Night-Rider," lines 16–17.

"On Being Ill"

VIRGINIA WOOLF

Considering how common illness is, how tremendous the spiritual change that it brings, how astonishing, when the lights of health go down, the undiscovered countries that are then disclosed, what wastes and deserts of the soul a slight attack of influenza brings to view, what precipices and lawns sprinkled with bright flowers a little rise of temperature reveals, what ancient and obdurate oaks are uprooted in us by the act of sickness, how we go down into the pit of death and feel the waters of annihilation close above our heads and wake thinking to find ourselves in the presence of the angels and the harpers when we have a tooth out and come to the surface in the dentist's arm-chair and confuse his "Rinse the mouth—rinse the mouth" with the greeting of the Deity stooping from the floor of Heaven to welcome us—when we think of this, as we are so frequently forced to think of it, it becomes strange indeed that illness has not taken its place with love and battle and jealousy among the prime themes of literature.

Deliverance

KEVIN CROSSLEY-HOLLAND

My skull cracks open.
Look at the birds,
looks at the birds released, a spray,
a fantail flowering.

First, the lark, up, out and away,
hitting top C like a piano-tuner;
the humming-bird, the mocking bird,
the bird of paradise;
look at the sparrows and pippets;
the gull like a longing,
sea-ranger never satisfied;
ravens, two of them,
heavy with the weight of Thought and Memory.

This is the day of the rainbow,
the bird with a twig in its beak.
At last, when least expected,
this is the great escape.
Uncontainable
they fly purposive, interweaving;
they mingle and they sing,
and I shall not go mad.

A Brain Wider Than the Sky

ANDREW LEVY

But if God or the central nervous system wants to punch me in the side of the face, or plant a warped kaleidoscopic vision where I should be seeing half a stop sign, there's nothing I can do about it, nothing I want to do about it, nothing left to do about it, but gape (in a metaphysical sense, of course) at the wonder of it all. That is the migrainy worldview: the migraines scour you, humble you, then they make you all dreamy and a sensation junkie, stuck in an imminent future tense always a little more alive than you ever desired, a memorable place if not a beautiful one, a place to build, if one can build castles in air. And I believe I can now, and I thank the headaches for that. This is a story about pain, the great, cowardly indescribable. But joined to that pain, rising from it like a phoenix, it is also a story about hope—hope blasted, then hope twisted, and then, finally just hope.

February 22: a new snowfall the night before, three inches or so, icy cold so the flakes don't cohere, they just sit on the ground like a coat of fur. We have strayed inside, blinds partially drawn, so when I walk outside with Aedan—he to move toy bulldozers and snowplows through the new snow and admire the tracks they make—I am completely blinded, my eyes long to shut, and even before I can shut them, I feel the visual world go dark with shafts and nodes of phosphorescence. I turn around, go inside, find a pair of sunglasses, blue and wraparound, and come back outside, but now, a different sensation: I am, I think, about seven feet tall. I am keenly aware of a new angle on things, a strange outburst of length in my calves and thighs. It lasts for about fifteen minutes. At first, I want to rebel against it, but then I think, why not, it's no stranger than the strangeness of snow and sunlight and no less natural.

Aedan has surprised us lately with some interesting news: he sees "colors" in front of his eyes, whether his eyes are open or closed, and only "sometimes." He says: "I see yellow here and here and here and here and here and here and here and here and here and here and here and here and here and here," as his finger points in the air at one place and then another, or draws a wavy or zigzagging line in space.

He says that he sees pictures, too: "a brachiosaurus herd," or his painted hand, and not all of it—only "here and here and here," and here he is touching parts of my hand to demonstrate what parts of his hand are visible: just the tips of the fingers. Aura, maybe: maybe he'll be a silly billy after all. Fifty-fifty. If so, he's already better at describing it than me, and I had a forty-year start. If not—well, it's hard to say where his imagination stops and his vision starts. It's harder to say it matters.

I ask him if he ever gets a headache. He says, "Once." "For how long?" I ask. "What is that time between a second and a minute?" he asks back.

I ask him if he likes seeing the colors, and he says very much. He also says he can see God sometimes: an old man in a red shirt and blue pants, long gray beard, a cane, and a friendly face, like "a straight line."

What is the job of the father here? Not much, I think. Show him for ropes, all the ropes, if he needs them. That's what this book is for, in case you hadn't guessed. But what else? Why tell him what he already knows?

The Hours

MICHAEL CUNNINGHAM

The headache is always there, waiting, and her periods of freedom, however long, always feel provisional. Sometimes the headache simply takes partial possession for an evening or a day or two, then withdraws. Sometimes it remains and increases until she herself subsides. At those times the headache moves out of her skull and into the world. Everything glows and pulses. Everything is infected with brightness, throbbing with it, and she prays for dark the way a wanderer lost in the desert prays for water. The world is every bit as barren of darkness as a desert is of water. There is no dark in the shuttered room, no dark behind her eyelids. There are only greater and lesser digress of radiance. . . . Eventually, when enough hours have passed, she emerges bloodied, trembling, but full of vision and ready, once she's rested, to work again. She dreads her lapses into pain and light and she suspects they are necessary. She has been free for quite some time now, for years. She knows how suddenly the headache can return but she discounts it in Leonard's presence, acts more firmly healthy that she sometimes feels. She will return to London. Better to die raving mad in London than evaporate in Richmond.

Morning

ROY FULLER

Through half-drawn curtains distant roses' daub
And a young blackbird, sepia still his prow,
Taking the berries of a berberis,
Each a pythagorean proposition
    Of angle, orb and tangents.

The iteration of the seasons must
Bring to me worsening health and history—
Such thoughts I waken to when noises hidden
In daytime wail far off or overhead
    Creak like John Gabriel Borkman.

And yet how raw one stays. I've never heard
Pronounced the word 'raceme' and look it up.
So much I've never read or heard. Perhaps
Some Spring within my reach will flower my long
    Unflowering wisteria.

As animals stagger up, amelioration
Of human ailments leads to ready tears
Of feeling for art and for the lives of others
And to activity in the noddle one thought
    Had ossified forever.

This early Summer morning the aperture
Beneath the oriented bedroom door—
And even its keyhole—are incandescent with
The sun in the still somewhat shady room of nights,
    Thrilling as light in childhood.

What a startling notion, really against the whole
Philosophy of what I've always thought of
As pessimistic life, that the end may be
Felicity: ianthine blossoming
    For fitter and unfried scions.

Night and Sunrise

ALAN BROWNJOHN

The cog-wheel abrasions are at it again
On this first glinting day of March,
Swerving over any pale surface, fastening
Blips of a crazed illumination on
The carpet, the walls, the half-typed page.

So again the old half-humorous yearning starts,
For the life of the darker months:
The sunless heavens, the easy velvet hours
When action soothes, and shadow onto shadow
Glides for a shadow satisfaction.

And truly, the heart of the educationist
Rises in autumn, as the dead leaves drift
Round blocks of switched-on light in heated rooms;
The colours of his season moderate
The strident freshness on those shoots of green . . .

But reproached one late June day, when she maintained
'Dark nights, cold weather, cold women,
Those are what you seem to want!' I tried to say
'Exegesis is difficult in summer, who
Can sort out the words from the spaces

'In a book read out of doors? Besides, your sun
Irradiates only the outer sides,
And deep down things the dearest darkness lives,
Where profundity waits to be dug for'
—When she put my book aside, and we went indoors

Discussing my eyesight and my character,
Lamenting or happy that the nights were already
Drawing in, and she closed the curtains.
              Who had won
I couldn't tell; but I was very glad she stayed
To try the night, and see the dawn up for me.

The Night-Rider

GAVIN EWART

The rider is not clear;
is it a man or a woman?
It could be a woman.
It is night. But is it night?
There are these painful lightnings
that fill the head.
There is nausea.

The conscientious rider
rides through the night
and the sickness of the night.
An axe is splitting the skull.
The rider rides.

The rider knows the eyes
will see again, calm;
that the axe will lose its edge.
The solution is partly
to keep on riding.

If you ride long enough
you come to sunrise,
to a gentle, natural light
that could hurt nobody,
sunshine and birdsong.

Half-Skull Days

ANNA LEAHY

Last week, it rained six days straight, not *for* six days straight, as it can back home in the Midwest, but *on* six consecutive days. In the eighteen months we have lived in Southern California we had not experienced more than a day of rain at a time, just a few showers over the course of more than a year. In the hills, there were evacuations and mudslides. On the coast, just thirty minutes away, a cliff was shearing off under two apartment buildings. CNN spent an hour on an effort to save a dog. Eventually, a rescue worker was lowered from a helicopter into the viaduct to wrestle with the dog and then, dog in his arms, be pulled back up to safety. The story ended well, but it might not have.

For that week, because of the repeated storms hitting the West Coast, accompanied by low barometric pressure, I worked to stave off migraine. I didn't succumb to the lure of bed. I never reached the point of no return, when I must be horizontal and still and in the dark and quiet, with an ice pack to my neck, for hours. When I become what Joan Didion, in her essay "In Bed," describes as "insensible to the world around me." Last week was a victory not possible a few years ago. Somehow, I've figured out how to live with migraine. It's taken research and trial and error, but I've managed to thrive despite migraine, perhaps even with it. I have become a migraineur, a connoisseur of migraine, in the original sense of *connoisseur* as being well acquainted with. This word connotes appreciation, too, which is an unexpected possibility.

That's not to say that staving off a migraine is not its own discomfort. A lurking migraine makes one off kilter, unwell. Like Didion, "I used to think that I could rid myself of this error by simply denying it, character over chemistry." Ignoring or denying it doesn't work. In the next stage of my migraine life, I thought that I could rid myself of this anomaly by actively fighting it, but one cannot eliminate migraine. So, staving off is the best I can do. Still, the lurking migraine is much better than the pain, nausea, and severe disorientation, all of it at once. Given the alternative, I'm thankful for the lurking migraine, even as I'm discouraged and not myself.

The moderate disorientation I felt last week is a result either of the underlying migraine waiting for me to turn attention away so that it can lurch within me or of the abortive medication, or both. But what caused the migraine itself is a tricky thing, as if it stays a step ahead. My migraines have instigators, which the medical literature appropriately calls *triggers. Bang* indeed! A hormone drop or weather front is what I call a *primary trigger,* though the official literature doesn't make this distinction among instigators. Either a hormone drop or a storm front can, and almost always does, cause a migraine.

Then there are *secondary triggers,* which must pair up or clump together to meet some secret threshold: freshly cut grass; mint, especially spearmint or anything mint-smelling in a green package; onions, especially on the breath hours later, but sometimes even as I cut them fresh, if I'm already in trouble; garlic, again especially garlic breath, which I can sometimes smell at a distance; certain flowers, though I don't know exactly which ones, beyond lilacs; lack of enough sleep, though what is enough varies; waiting too long to eat, a trigger I share with my aunt; wine; dehydration; stress or, rather, the slide out of stress. Perhaps, some of the smells are not so much triggers as they are evidence of aura, my hypersensitivity to stimuli I would otherwise not notice. It's a distinction I make: when I'm hypersensitive, the unpleasant smell of spearmint is a trigger, makes things worse, but the vibrant greens in the landscape is aura, a pleasant precursor to pain.

Part of migraine prevention, I know through experience, is avoiding these triggers. But there is no avoiding weather and hormones. Andrew Levy, in his book *A Brain Wider Than the Sky,* points out, "While two-thirds of women with migraines identify menstruation as a cause, only 15 percent have migraines *only* during menstruation, complicating the chain of cause and effect." While I don't have migraine *only* during my period, it *always* brings me to migraine, so the causal relationship doesn't seem that complicated to me. My gynecologist nodded knowingly. She told me to skip the seven sugar pills at the end of the contraceptive's circle, to jump ahead to the next pack instead of swallowing the *off* week, so that I could schedule a migraine for every nine weeks or so. There's a good deal of information available about migraine: medical studies and personal anecdotes, in print and online at sites like WebMD and My Migraine Connection. Perhaps because I've had so much schooling, sorting through what's out there and figuring out how it applies to me is part of understanding my headache-plagued self.

Levy writes, "Roughly 60 percent of all migraineurs identify weather change as a trigger, but half of those identify the wrong weather change, blaming falling barometric pressure when they should blame rising, or a cold blast when it's dry air they should vilify." What unsettled me when I first read this is that when I sought treatment from my general practitioner a few years ago, she said, *Really, weather? I've never heard of that, but if you say so.* Because the experience of migraine is individualized, each of us with different triggers or symptoms, our patterns often shifting, the menstruation and weather-change percentages seem near-consensus to me. How had my physician not known weather could be a trigger, if the majority of sufferers identify it as such? That we blame the wrong weather phenomenon strikes me as a lack of knowledge of meteorological terminology, rather than a lack of knowledge of our own bodies. In the Midwest, for instance, a cold blast is often accompanied by dry air, which is compounded by turning up the furnace.

One of the unexpected benefits of moving to Southern California, as opposed to the Midwest, is the lack of weather here and, therefore, migraine prevention, although locals dispute this lack-of-weather claim. Joan Didion, in her "Los Angeles Notebook," writes, "Easterners commonly complain that there is no 'weather' at all in Southern California, that the days and the seasons slip by relentlessly, numbingly bland. That is quite misleading." Having just been through a week of rain, I see her point and admit my narrow definition. But to say there is weather here is somewhat misleading to me. Any seasonal shift in Southern California is subtle compared with the fire-red autumns and blizzard winters of my childhood.

For the first year here, time stood almost still, each day pretty much like the last, the various flowering bushes taking turns blooming all year long. It creates a pleasantly bewildering state of mind. A day still felt roughly like twenty-four hours, but the larger timeframes became less discernible, less meaningful. My changed sense of time—my diminished ability to perceive time moving forward over weeks and months—diminished my ability to perceive stress. If tomorrow will be much like today, what's the hurry? As much as I miss sitting on a warm radiator to watch big snowflakes fall, I am awestruck that a change in geography can have such a profoundly positive effect on me, that the Midwest I adore kicked the legs out from under me, while the geography I cannot grasp allows me to see the light of every day. Strange medicine, sunshine.

My secondary triggers are not always, or individually, problems. They work like genre: if you have a character in a cowboy hat, you don't necessarily have a Western, but if John Wayne wearing a cowboy hat pulls his gun at the saloon, then you probably do. Of course, you can have a Western without John Wayne. So, prevention becomes a quest for clues, for awareness of exactly how the self rubs up against the world in a given moment. I have become better at noticing the familiar stranger as soon as he rides into town. I can look at a pack of spearmint gum now and know whether it might be a trigger today, or whether it's temporarily benign to me.

The staved-off migraine's disorientation has left me aware of my own incoherence, my inability to track time accurately or to guess what I might say next, or not be able to say. When I couldn't think of the word *scale,* upon which I had slammed my toe and made a racket in the bathroom only moments before, I pantomimed stepping onto the scale and looking down to see my weight. But even my husband is not used to this sort of communication and shrugged; at least he was no longer worried that I'd injured myself. I would not call what I felt in this semi-articulate moment *pain,* but I was suffering. Every bit of coherence I mustered took great effort, when lucidity is usually taken for granted, like breathing.

Even after the fact, as I try to articulate what I feel exactly, in the staving off or in the depths of a full-blown migraine, I fall short. *Depths,* in fact, is the wrong word, for it implies direction. There exists no word for the feeling of simultaneously being boxed in and without any boundary. Levy writes, "Maybe the language of migraine is a run-on sentence, in part because you can't ever find the right words, in part because the migraine is also a compound of too many interlocking features." Yes. Exactly. When I read someone else's account of migraine, it rings true. But it's also wrong. I think fragments, too, are the language of migraine: a subject slipping out of grammatical grasp, a period interrupting a thought's completion. The language of incoherence, piecemeal thinking. Or being felled in your tracks.

Or, as Levy goes on, "Maybe the language of migraine isn't really language at all. It's language just disappearing." If that's true, what does that mean for the migraineur who is a writer? If the migraineur's language is just disappearing, how does Didion put so much carefully organized language on the page?

Because I was so conscious of the migraine beneath my surface this past week, I expected to be unproductive—and, in fact, felt sluggish in the moment and in the moment I expected next. Instead, though, I finished drafting a short story that had lodged in my head on a plane ride a few weeks earlier, the longest story I have ever written and the first story I have written in years. And I wrote, from scratch to an unwieldy whole, an essay about marriage. These writings may be no good, in the end, for migraine skews my judgment, making me both overly enamored and utterly disappointed with given things.

I also participated successfully in two meetings on Tuesday, though I may have inadvertently offended a colleague at the first because my wording was territorial or my tone was strident, so I patched up that possibility with an e-mail afterward. Sometimes, I say things without thinking or don't remember what I've just said, though I know I've said something. There's no predicting the next migraine conversation, even in hindsight.

I edited an interview my students had done, and I scoured through a new website to generate a four-page list of corrections before it launched. With an actual migraine, a full-blown headache, I could not have looked directly at a computer screen without keeling over. Often, the stark contrast of black type on white paper is too much, or I read a line again and again until it becomes a knife in my eyes. Last week, I even went to the post office, where the ceiling fan strobes make me queasy even on good days, and to the grocery store. I was, overall, incredibly productive. I didn't hurry as if I faced a deadline, though I had the sense that time was running out—and still running out. I kept doing merely one more thing before the pain knocked me over, but the pain stayed just at bay.

So, I came to terms with that migraine. But it has not always been that way, and I've been trying to figure out why and, by extension, what role migraine plays in my life.

I don't remember my first migraine. They began less than ten years ago, I know, but I did not not the first one because I defined it as migraine only a few years later, once I became aware that my headaches fit the pattern. I remember one migraine that developed during a meeting about reinstating the Illinois Poet Laureate, a position that had been held for decades by Gwendolyn Brooks and, before her, Carl Sandburg. On the way into Chicago, the world could not have been more vibrant, every line sharp, every color crisp, my body filled with energy. I could hear the crisp conversations of others on the El, their individual inflections. I perceived everything; I soaked in the world through my senses. I felt great—really great—for no logical reason. Back then, I did not recognize aura for what it was: a prelude.

Forty minutes into the meeting, after most of the important discussion was accomplished, both disorientation and pain hit. This initial transition is slower but akin to when *The Wizard of Oz* switches from black-and-white to color, only in reverse. I wanted to lie down flat. The earth's spin dizzied me. I felt I might fly off the earth's surface. Or I was growing too heavy to move far. I wondered how I would make it home. I knew I *had* to get home. Outside, in the oppressive air that precedes a large Midwestern storm, I made my first certain connection between the cause of my pain and the migraine itself and also between the beautiful aura and the horrible pain. Yet, the next time the world was vibrant, I didn't make the connection; the pain took me by surprise again and again, the aura remaining an ingenious ruse for years.

I remember another migraine that developed on a flight from Chicago to Oregon. I could barely walk from the plane. I wanted to press my head against a cold hard surface that had no odor of its own. I wanted to spit out the words on my tongue. But the thought of moving my mouth—no. I crawled into bed, waking every few hours to hear my sister and my husband celebrate Thanksgiving. I did not believe that I would ever get out of bed. I concentrated on seconds at a time. I could not imagine a future.

Migraine hasn't killed me, though. In fact, it ebbs and flows in ways that make it manageable, often hitting the day after a big event—like the final grading before that trip to Oregon—or lurking while I teach a class. I tend to be most pathetic only when I can afford to be. Like a parasite, it can't kill its host; it requires a level of thriving in me to sustain the pattern and variation that is its goal.

Because they often occur in the immediate aftermath of heightened activity or demands, for a long time I called them *tension headaches* and blamed them entirely on stress. Didion writes of the "migraine personality," which seems a perfect crucible for stress: "ambitious, inward, intolerant of error, rather rigidly organized, perfectionist." I don't keep a perfect house or give great attention to my own appearance. I have to remind myself to comb my hair at least once a day, and I don't always vacuum under the furniture, though I know I should. But I do have household rules—as for proper loading of the dishwasher or kitchen cabinet organization—which my husband struggles to value and, therefore, follow. A grammar error or a misinterpreted remark can stick in my craw like a popcorn kernel in a molar. These adjectives—*ambitious, inward, intolerant of error*—and the personality they represent don't describe the whole of us, but there's something that rings true. I have come to wonder whether this migraine personality is a contributing factor or whether certain personality traits become honed in response to migraine. The qualities may, after all, be excellent ways to deal with migraine. If my cabinets are in order, I can find a can of soup or the icepack in the freezer door on a day in which I become insensible, in which a squint is too open-eyed, too tense. If my world is well ordered, it will cohere when I do not. The migraine personality as precondition too simply puts the blame on me as the *cause* of my condition, as if I could cure myself by mixing up the glassware and plates on the same cabinet shelf, as if no blithe spirit could be afflicted, or as if pain is punishment for ambition.

Family history may be somewhat more useful than personality in understanding my condition: my maternal grandmother, maternal aunt, and sister all suffered migraines long before I did. My grandmother didn't call them *migraines,* or even *headaches,* perhaps because she thought headaches were associated with hangovers. No, she was *under the weather* or *not feeling well,* and she couldn't take naps because she'd awaken in pain. My grandmother had a stroke in a taxicab, coming home from the dentist, so I worry about stroke, even though my cholesterol numbers are very good. Some studies indicate that migraineurs are twice as likely to have a stroke and that more than a quarter of the strokes in people under forty-five years of age are caused by or correlated with migraine. Migraineurs with aura are more likely than those without aura to suffer a stroke, and migraineurs on the Pill who smoke are at even higher risk. At least, I've never smoked; in fact, the thought of a cigarette with a migraine makes me queasy. The tricky distinction between causation and correlation matters, but isn't often made by researchers.

Unlike my grandmother and aunt, my mother isn't sure she's ever had a headache in her life, a thing I have trouble imagining. She deals with her own pain, the result of clubfoot and the childhood surgeries that allowed her to walk. But she thinks of a headache as an on-or-off state, not a condition, a thing you might have once for some reason and maybe never again, like chicken pox, or something acute, but swiftly healed, like stubbing your toe. She doesn't doubt it's painful, but she doesn't understand it.

Even if a given personality and heredity explain migraine, that information is a crapshoot and not a cure. My mother-in-law swears she can avert a headache by pinching pressure points near her knee as soon as she feels it coming on. That didn't work for me, either because I don't recognize a migraine early enough or don't press my thumb and forefinger hard enough or in exactly the right places. A friend's mother attests to biofeedback. Another trick is to, at the migraine's first twinkling, plunge your hands under the hottest water you can stand.

Mostly, though, for cures we turn to medicine. There exist two types of medication: preventative and abortive. Preventative meds are recommended for someone with more than one migraine a week and include a host of drugs used to treat other conditions. If you have asthma—and one study indicates you're twice as likely to have asthma if you have migraine—you shouldn't take beta blockers; channel blockers have a lot of drug interactions; antidepressants have side effects and can interact with abortive migraine meds; and anti-seizure and allergy drugs can leave you too drowsy to accomplish more than if you'd had the migraine. In many cases, no one knows why these drugs prevent migraine, and they are hit and miss at reducing either frequency or severity. Prevention is as much a crapshoot as causation, so I've not yet tried these treatments. They represent an admission and commitment for which I must not be ready.

For a while, aspirin, if I took it the day before a storm or my period was coming, helped take the edge off, a sort of mild prevention. Now, I resort to abortive pills. The expensive one works okay. Even with insurance, it costs $70 for six tablets, and I often have to take more than one pill because I use the lower dose. The cheaper one seems to work better, and I probably want it to. Without insurance, it would cost more than $250 for nine tablets, but with insurance, it is $10. The tablet must be taken at first onset, before I'm sure the inkling will actually become a migraine. With the more expensive medication, I hesitated, telling myself I didn't want to overmedicate, didn't want to take it just in case. I'm surprised at how my risk assessment has adjusted in relation to cost. Now, I act quickly, popping that pill if I can think of anything that might have triggered my migrainy inkling.

The last time I took this pill, though, I felt as if I had the worst hangover of my life. My intestinal tract twitched, my neck grew sore and wobbly, my throat swelled, my whole self was physically uneasy. It wasn't worse than my worst migraine; I could function, just barely. But it was worse than having the sort of migraine I now usually have; the reaction scared me, in part because I didn't expect it, in part because it didn't get better as the day eased on. Just when I'd thought I'd figured some things out about migraine, this reaction took me by surprise with a new version. Migraine would not be outdone. I could not let myself sleep when I felt so unfamiliar.

My experience and history with migraine is not exactly the same as Didion's, nor does it sync up point by point with Levy's, but reading them, I felt as if I were among familiar company. When I read "In Bed" for the first time eighteen months ago, after several friends recommended it, I immediately felt relief that someone else understood and could put migraine into words. Even though there existed differences among our experiences, I was excited when I read the descriptions of *my* migraines in Didion's work. *Yes, someone understands!* Finally, reading that—and other information and others' descriptions—made me feel better about my lot in life. I was not alone in this migraine thing; my experience was validated by their experiences.

Two weeks later, I looked at the essay again and noticed its publication date. I was dumbfounded: it had been published more than forty years ago. Why was my experience with migraine little better than in the late 1960s? Why had so little been done since, in *Bewitched*, Darrin's persnickety, rigidly organized, even perfectionist, mortal mother complained of *sick headaches* triggered by the stress of witnessing witchcraft, of brushing up against the world in an unexpected, illogical way? We have a great deal of collective information, but that hasn't changed the individual, very human experience of migraine.

If that's the case, I thought, Hildegard of Bingen, who suffered migraine in the twelfth century, is as good a touchstone as Didion. Of course, Hildegard didn't define her aura and pain as migraine; it was contemporary writer and neurologist Oliver Sacks and others who have made that diagnosis. No, Hildegard defined her migraine symptoms as visions and signs from God and, driven by them, became a prolific writer and composer, headed up two convents, offered medical advice, and eventually joined the Canon of Saints. Given her hefty and numerous accomplishments, I imagine she probably had a so-called migraine personality.

Aura, if we look to Hildegard, is the gift of an altered state. Even beyond aura, when she was bedridden, she managed to use her condition as leverage, claiming she had been stricken because God was unhappy that the abbot refused to let her nuns move to a more independent convent. She turned *woe is me* into *it's your fault*. Instead of letting it do her in, Hildegard somehow—using the conventions of her time—gave her migraine purpose and defined it within the context of her own ambitions. There exists great danger in women accepting their plights, talking of their afflictions as blessings. I'm uncomfortable with the idea that one should be grateful for suffering.

Several years ago, a dear friend, who also shares a deep interest in Hildegard but does not share migraine, wrote that she was suffering from writer's block. Maybe I didn't fully appreciate my friend's excruciating pain when I wrote back that writer's block might be a natural or useful part of the larger process. By that, I meant that perhaps we need, in some deeply physiological way or in some mysterious cognitive way, to shore up. My friend continues to be an exceptionally productive writer overall, and I believed then that her words would flow again, that she would reach a point of ah-hah when words would fall back into place for her and out onto the page. It's called the bathtub moment—or eureka—based on an anecdote about Archimedes, who had worked and worked on a problem, only to be struck with the solution as he stepped into his bath and saw the water level rise. Though that story is likely made up, Einstein had eureka moments in the midst of his intellectual daydreaming, after intense mathematical work. Cognitive scientists assert that incubation—which can feel like an impasse—and eureka are important stages in the creative process. But my comments sounded to my blocked friend like dismissal of the severity of her problem. My words hurt her, or compounded her hurting.

I continue to struggle to understand the relationship between writing and suffering. Clearly, acute suffering itself is unproductive. One of Nancy Andreasen's interesting points in *The Creating Brain* is that, while chronic, non-episodic mental illness like schizophrenia is debilitating, some mental illnesses, like mood disorders, involve sensitivity to stimuli that may be akin to aspects of creativity. That's not to say that mental illness is creativity, but that the two states may share some characteristics. It strikes me that migraine, too, is an episodic experience of over-sensitivity to stimuli. *The world is too much.* Mood disorders—and alcoholism, perhaps to dampen the mood swings—appear more common in writers, but the writers in Andreasen's study "indicated that they were unable to be creative when either depressed or manic." Conclusions based on small studies and on anecdotal lore seem a bit loosey-goosey to me, but what if short periods of utter lack of creativity—whether from migraine, writer's block, or depression—are part of a larger process that *is* greatly productive? What if some aspects of the unproductive period, like sensitivity to external stimuli or physical self-awareness or obsessive thinking, are strange, alternative—destructive—versions of some attributes of creative productivity?

The onset of my first migraines coincides with my increased success as a writer—publication and productivity—rather than signaling a stalling point. I cannot possibly attest to causation, as I had undoubtedly reached, after numerous years, a point in my career and in my writing practice that allowed for important strides and external recognition. It is possible, too, that learning to manage migraine and developing an awareness of my physical self in relation to my surroundings may encourage the kind of discipline I need for writing. To embrace and credit migraine for my creative work would be ludicrous. Even if it plays a role, other things matter much more; Andreasen mentions intellectual freedom, a community of creative people, fair competition, mentors, and economic stability.

But what if migraine matters in the way Didion suggests: "For when the pain recedes, ten or twelve hours later, everything goes with it, all the hidden resentments, all the vain anxieties. The migraine has acted as a circuit breaker, and the fuses have emerged intact. There is a pleasant convalescent euphoria." Migraine, because it debilitates, forces a temporary letting go; I can't hang onto much when in the throes of its pain. In its wake, though, migraine offers a couple of days of exhilarated awareness or relief or calm before one moves back into the world as it usually is. Perhaps, also, I feel the need to accomplish something before the next migraine comes to shoot me in the back before I hear its spurs jingling. I'm usually not sure when that next migraine will be, but I expect it to come. I have an unknown timeframe between migraines and can't procrastinate.

Given what I now know about migraine, how might it fit into my creative process? Hildegard did not write immediately about her visions, but eventually was, by her own admission, compelled by illness to set her hand to writing. My poem "Barbie Gets a Migraine," which I posted online at My Migraine Connection, sorts through my circumstances by afflicting a perfect plastic version. Certainly, plenty of people experience the altered state of aura or the excruciating pain of headache, but are not compelled to write metered verse, compose piano sonatas, or paint cubist portraits. Writers don't need migraines; anyone would be far better off without them. But if we're stuck with these migraines, maybe we can figure out how not to let them disrupt life entirely or permanently.

I'd like to go further; I'd like to construe them as useful, despite how uncomfortable I am with claiming that disorientation or pain is something for which I should feel lucky. Levy suggests that a person can be "smart and kind enough to respect their value." It seems that every migraineur I read about—Didion, Levy, Hildegard, Emily Dickinson, Picasso, Thomas Jefferson—reached a point at which he or she said, *okay, I give up. Now I must acknowledge this part of myself and get to my work.* Migraine "entwines itself with a life and with the purpose of the life," Levy writes. "But to understand this fact, I soon learned, meant thinking in narrative terms, about a whole life, not in episodes." When I have a full-blown migraine, it defines me. It consumes me, and I am only that migrained body—not a writer, not a teacher, not a friend, not a wife—while it lasts. But migraine is episodic, which invites me to experience the condition as part of my larger life story.

There are always several ways to perceive a given event or to tell a particular narrative. My lawyer-parents taught me early on that it is better to have many witnesses to an accident you cause than to have only one. Many witnesses—Didion, Levy, Hildegard—will provide the jury with many versions of the migraine. And the jury itself may come up with a dozen ways of sorting through those stories.

That dog rescued from the rising flood waters last week presented rescue workers with two choices: let the dog find his own way to safety (or fail to do so), or risk their own lives to save the dog. The fire fighters could be passive or active. From my vantage, at home lounging in a comfy chair, the dog looked to be in no immediate danger of being swept away. The rescue team chose to rescue the dog, but they claimed it wasn't because dogs are worth rescuing. They said that they risked their lives because they feared, if they didn't, someone less well trained would, thereby necessitating a more desperate rescue of a human being. They'd seen that before;

they knew how badly things could go. So, they looked at the big picture, considered the best use of their resources, and trusted their expertise. They understood human nature and drew from past experience. And yes, maybe Joe St. Georges, the man lowered from the helicopter to grab the dog, has a soft spot for animals, too. We try to figure out what we can do so that our story—or at least the episode in which we're currently immersed—ends well. Or at least, we try to ensure that things don't get worse. People will disagree whether it's the right decision.

I have come to think of migraine not as a constant, lurking threat, though it is that. I have come to understand it not as something that can be denied or fought, though it can be treated. Instead, migraine is part of the story I must tell of who am I now. Part of what tells my story. All the research, documentation, and anecdotes are right, but they aren't all right at the same time, not from every vantage. I will be grateful if menopause makes migraine part of my past history, though I fear it could become worse. Unlike Levy, I know I can live without it. I want to live without it.

As Hildegard might have said and as Didion says by the end of her essay, "I am wise in its ways . . . I count my blessings." Unlike the rescue workers, who wavered between action and inaction, who had a decision to make, I have no choice about these extremes, little control over the way events unfold within these extreme states. That said, sorting through the available information and others' accounts of migraine, along with accumulating my own experience of it, has taught me a way to live as a migraineur.

An old term for the condition came from the Greek word for *half skull*. Sometimes during migraine, I press my hand over the eye where the pain is gathering and imagine the dark and the pressure of my hand replacing that side of my head. No one wishes to be left with half a skull. But sometimes, I have only half a skull with which to live.

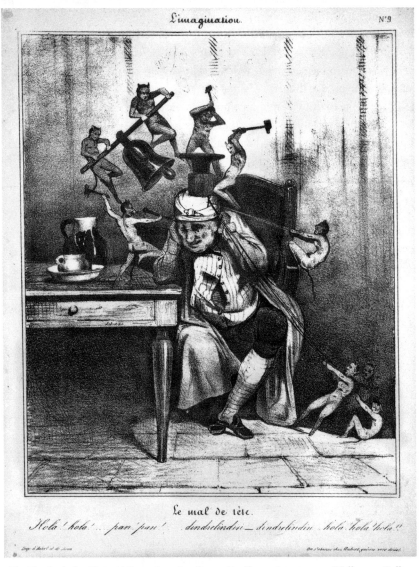

Permissions Acknowledgments

JANE AUSTEN: "On a Headache," in *The Works of Jane Austen*. Vol. 6. *Minor Works*. Ed. R. W. Chapman. New York: Oxford University Press, 1954.

LAURIE BISCONTI: "A Patient's Perspective: A Friend Like No Other." *Headache: The Journal of Head and Face Pain* (1961), http://onlinelibrary.wiley.com/journal/10.1111/ (ISSN) 1526–4610; permission conveyed through Copyright Clearance Center, Inc.

ANITA BROOKNER: Excerpt from *A Misalliance* by Anita Brookner, copyright 1986 by Selobrook Ltd. Used by permission of Pantheon Books, an imprint of the Knopf Double-day Publishing Group, a division of Penguin Random House LLC. All rights reserved. A. M. Heath & CO. LTD. Used by permission of A. M. Heath & Co. Ltd. London.

ALAN BROWNJOHN: "Night and Sunrise" in *Night and Sunrise. An Anthology of New Poems*, ed. John Lowbury. Aberystwyth, Dyfed, Wales: Celion Publishing, 1978. Repro-duced by kind permission of the author c/o by Rosica Colin Limited, London.

CATHERINE BUSH: *Claire's Head*. "Rachel's House of Pain," Copyright 2004. Reprinted by permission of Emblem/McClelland & Stewart, a division of Penguin Random House Canada Limited. All rights reserved. Excerpts from *Claire's Head* are copyright 2004 by Catherine Bush. Any third party use of this material, outside of this publication, is prohibited. Interested parties must apply directly to Penguin Random House Canada Limited for permission.

AMY CLAMPITT: "An Anatomy of Migraine" from *The Collected Poems of Amy Clampitt*, copyright 1997 by the Estate of Amy Clampitt. Used by permission of Alfred A. Knopf, an imprint of the Knopf Doubleday Publishing Group, a division of Penguin Random House LLC. All rights reserved.

KEVIN CROSSLEY-HOLLAND: "Deliverance" from *Times Oriel* by Kevin Crossley-Holland. Published by Hutchinson, 1983. Copyright Kevin Crossley-Holland. Repro-duced by permission of the author c/o Rogers, Coleridge & White Ltd., 20 Powis Mews, London W11 1JN.

MICHAEL CUNNINGHAM: Excerpt from *The Hours*. Copyright 1998 by Michael Cun-ningham. Reprinted by permission of Farrar, Straus and Giroux. Reprinted by permission of HarperCollins Publishers Ltd. Michael Cunningham 1998.

EMILY DICKINSON: "Pain Has an Element of Blank," *The Poems of Emily Dickinson: Reading Edition*, edited by Ralph W. Franklin, Cambridge, Mass.: The Belknap Press of Harvard University Press, Copyright © 1998, 1999 by the President and Fellows of Harvard College. Copyright © 1951, 1955 by the President and Fellows of Harvard College. Copyright © renewed 1979, 1983 by the President and Fellows of Harvard College.

EDWARD LOWBURY: "Hoof Beats in the Head," in *Night and Sunrise. An Anthology of New Poems* edited by Edward Lowbury. Aberystwyth, Dyfed, Wales: Celion Publishing, 1978. Reprinted with the permission of Ruth Lowbury.

HILARY MANTEL: Excerpt from *Giving up the Ghost. A Memoir.* New York: Picador, 2003. Reprinted by permission of Henry Holt and Company. All rights reserved.

GAIL MAZUR: "Dear Migraine." *Poets.org.* https://www.poets.org/poetsorg/poem/dear-migraine. Accessed December 15, 2018.

IMAN MERSAL: "I Describe a Migraine" in *Kenyon Review,* New Series, 28, no. 2 (Spring 2006). Permission is granted by the author.

BRADFORD MORROW: From *The Almanac Branch* by Bradford Morrow. Copyright 1991 by Bradford Morrow. Reprinted with the permission of Simon & Schuster, Inc. All rights reserved.

MICHAEL MORSE: *Void and Compensation [Migraine].* Marfa, Texas: Canarium Books, 2015. Permission is granted by the author.

MURIEL NELSON: "Sun and Migraine," *Beloit Poetry Journal* 57 no. 1 (Fall, 2006).

KATHLEEN J. O'SHEA: "I Know Upon Awakening," in *So Much More Than a Headache: Understanding Migraine through Literature.* Kent: Kent State University Press, 2020.

LINDA PASTAN: "Migraine," from *An Early Afterlife* by Linda Pastan. Copyright 1995 by Linda Pastan. Used by permission of W. W. Norton & Company, Inc. 1995 by Linda Pastan. Used by permission of Linda Pastan in care of the Jean V. Naggar Literary Agency, Inc. (permissions@jvnla.com).

OLIVER SACKS: "Patterns" from *Hallucinations* by Oliver Sacks, copyright © 2012 by Oliver Sacks. Used by permission of Alfred A. Knopf, an imprint of the Knopf Doubleday Publishing Group, a division of Penguin Random House LLC. All rights reserved.

OLIVER SACKS: Excerpt from *The River of Consciousness* by Oliver Sacks, compilation copyright 2017 by The Oliver Sacks Foundation. Used by permission of Alfred A. Knopf, an imprint of the Knopf Doubleday Publishing Group, a division of Penguin Random House LLC. All rights reserved. Used by permission of Penguin Random House Canada.

ELAINE SCARRY. *The Body in Pain.* New York: Oxford University Press, 1985.

JUDY Z. SEGAL. *Health and the Rhetoric of Medicine.* Carbondale: Southern Illinois University Press, 2008.

MAIA SEPP. *The Migraine Mafia.* Middletown: Lucky Bat Books, 2013. Permission is granted by the author.

JACK SHOLL, *Migraine: The Eternal Return.* Bloomington, Ind.: Author House, 2011.

ALBERT SANDS SOUTHWORTH AND JOSIAH JOHNSON Hawes. "Margaret Fuller." Ca. 1850. The Metropolitan Museum of Art. Image copyright © The Metropolitan Museum of Art. Image source: Art Resource, NY.

LISA GUSKIN-STONESTREET: "Six Explanations for Migraine," *Blackbird* 14, no. 1 (Spring 2015). Permission is granted by the author.

BRIAN TIERNEY: "Migraine," *The Gettysburg Review* 29:3 (Autumn 2016).

SALLIE TISDALE: "An Uncommon Pain." Copyright 2013 *Harper's Magazine.* All Rights reserved. Reproduced from the May issue by special permission.

JANE CAVE WINSCOM: "The Head-Ache," and "Written the First Morning of the Author's Bathing at Written the First Morning of the Author's Bathing at Teignmouth." 1786. *Poems on Various Subjects, Entertaining, Elegiac, and Religious.* The fourth edition, Bristol: Printed by N. Biggs, 1795. Public Domain.